LISTEN TO THE WISEST OF ALL

Listen to the Wisest of All

Rita Blockman

and

Kimberly Morin

Photography by
Charles Mercer

Elder Press
Champaign, Illinois

Listen to the Wisest of All
P.O. Box 6716
Champaign, IL 61826 USA

Visit our Web site at www.listentothewisest.com

• • •

Listen to the Wisest of All

Printed in the United States of America

First printing: September 2007
10 9 8 7 6 5 4 3 2 1

• • •

Library of Congress Cataloging-in-Publication Data
Listen to the Wisest of All
Listen to the Wisest of All / Rita Blockman & Kimberly Morin
p. cm.
2007902972
ISBN 978-0-9795024-0-8

• • •

Book and cover design: Paul Edwards, Midnight Graphics
Printed at Faulstich Printing, Danville, IL

• • •

PHOTO CREDITS
Charles Mercer

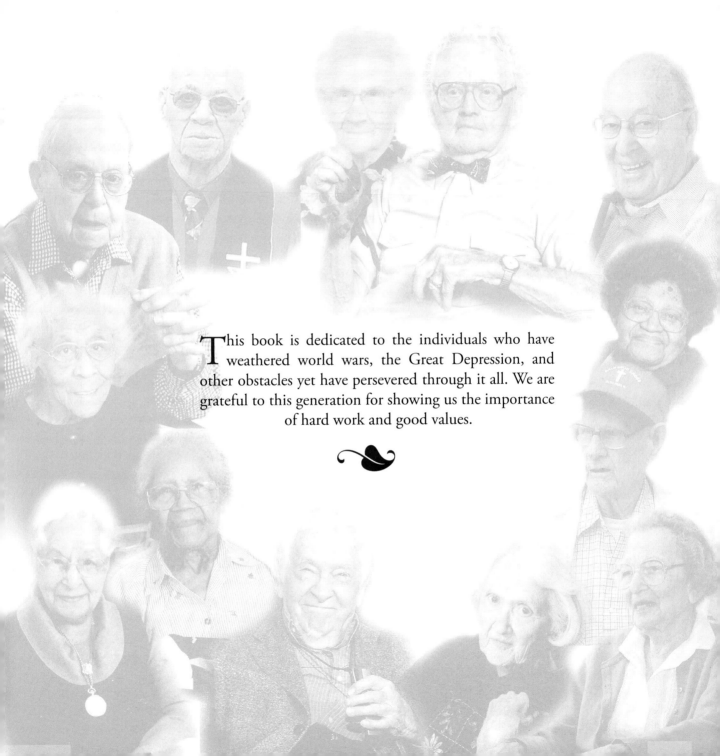

This book is dedicated to the individuals who have weathered world wars, the Great Depression, and other obstacles yet have persevered through it all. We are grateful to this generation for showing us the importance of hard work and good values.

PREFACE

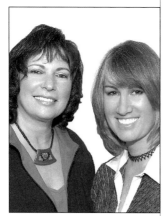

Rita   Kim

Our purpose in writing this book is to illustrate life through the retelling of the experiences of the many inspirational seniors we have interviewed. Most are over ninety years old and several are centenarians. They honestly and eagerly relayed to us their unique insights on a myriad of subjects, offering priceless wisdom of value to younger generations. The interviewees shared inspiring life stories, their strong spiritual beliefs, their advice to today's youth, and how all were deeply touched by friendship, poetry, music, or nature. Their recorded stories were written as vignettes that reveal the deeper nuances of life, love, and the passions that gave meaning to their lives. Each chapter is dedicated to one person or couple. Beautiful black-and-white photographs illustrate their stories. The dignity of these men and women, who share with us the wisdom that comes only from being fortunate enough to have lived a long life, is splendidly captured by these photographs.

We think that the timing of our book is fortunate, as it should appeal to baby boomers as well as many different types of populations in our society who would be extremely receptive to and interested in the unique perspective given by people who have lived almost a century (and in several cases even longer). There has been a resurgence of interest in preserving the legacies of those who have come before us. In response, college courses are now teaching how to write stories that capture the wisdom shared by the elderly population. The vignettes we have written represent people from different ethnicities who articulate their thoughts on their varied philosophies of life, unique histories, and daily activities. We feel that, although there are many books in the inspirational and spiritual genre, the concept of this book is markedly different. The intimate stories of so many exceptional individuals, enhanced by sensitive photographic images, will engage and reward the thoughtful reader who is searching for meaning and direction in facing today's complex challenges.

ACKNOWLEDGMENTS

Our book would never have been completed without the support and encouragement of a number of people. We wish to express our deepest gratitude to all the seniors we interviewed in the preparation of this book.

We particularly want to thank Hilda Banks for her professionalism, her continued support, and for the many hours she contributed to the editing of this book. She truly cared about the project and what we were trying to accomplish.

We also greatly appreciate the initial editing and support provided by Krista Kruse and Jeanine Berlocher, dear friends. Thanks also to Kallie Norton and Katie Carmody for their immeasurable contributions.

Special thanks go to our photographer, Charles Mercer, who provided us with creative and insightful pictures of our interviewees. Likewise, our graphic artist, Paul Edwards, amazed us with his artistic abilities.

We could not have accomplished anything without the love and support of our families—husbands Arnie and Todd; our children Rachel and Jonathan; Danielle and Hannah; and Kim's parents, Dan and Carol Snyder.

Many other family members, dear friends and acquaintances took the time to read our stories, and several of them provided us with excellent suggestions. These family members and friends include Rita's sister Ellen, Kim's brother Bryan, Barb Vabic, Cyndie Norton, Gloria Valenti, Bob Griffith, Anita and Steve Hamburg, Rose Vabic, Eddie Brandt, Judith Seligman, Kimm Allen, Brandi Allen, Michelle Butsch, Deb Williams, Sten Johansen, Elizabeth Jackson, Aparna Rahman, Vida Mazzocco, Annice Taft, and Patricia Edwards. Thanks to the Wilson, Trenkamp, and Michalos families for their friendship and support.

A number of individuals, including the William Gingold family, Representative Tim Johnson, Bill Houlihan, Sharon Bowen, Tim Mitchell, Dennis Donaldson, and Jennifer Hess, provided us with invaluable contacts.

Finally, this book is a lasting testament to the authors' long friendship through the best and worst of times.

To Lilly: who faithfully stayed beside Rita during the writing of this book.

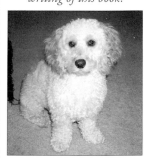

INTRODUCTION

We have always been told about the value of listening. Nevertheless, I didn't realize how profoundly my coauthor, Kim Morin, and I would be affected by listening to the inspirational stories that were told to us during the two-and-a-half-year period during which we gathered material and wrote this book. Kim and I met twenty years ago when she applied for a job in my office as an assistant. Several comments that she made during our interview impressed me, and there was a "realness" about her that I had never quite experienced before. We worked together for a few years, developed a productive working relationship, and became good friends. Even after Kim accepted another position, we still remained close.

The idea for the book originated from the experiences Kim had listening to the stories of her two grandmothers every summer. She remembers asking about their growing-up years, lives, and dreams. She never took notes and has relied on her memory to reflect on all the things she learned and treasures to this day. Kim regrets that all of the stories she heard were never written down. When she called me and asked if we could interview seniors who were close to ninety years of age or older, I was enthralled with the idea.

We immediately hired an extremely creative photographer, Charles Mercer, who had an uncanny ability to put our subjects at ease. He also was able to photograph each person in a way that captured the essence of their personalities. As Kim and I interviewed people, establishing a trusting relationship with each one, I soon realized that their stories, friendships, and advice on a wide variety of topics filled a void for me that I had so longed to satisfy during my life.

After continuously expressing ideas related to our book with friends and family throughout the community, we slowly acquired names of potential seniors to interview. Kim tape-recorded each interview and transcribed it verbatim. Additionally, we took extensive notes during some of our interviews. Written statements granting permission to publish were obtained from each individual. Although we interviewed more seniors for our project than are included here, we reduced the number of stories selected to include individuals from as many diverse walks of life and as wide a range of socio-economic status as possible.

We learned great life lessons from each person we interviewed, and many of the individuals expressed beliefs to us that were life-affirming. They also articulated emotions and ideas that we often felt and thought but couldn't put into words. We truly understand now what it means when people say that life is simply a matter of perspective. We will all inevitably face good and bad events in our lives. How we choose to look at things makes all the difference. Each person we developed a relationship with was dealing with some disability, whether it was navigating a wheelchair, utilizing a hearing device, walking with a cane, or overcoming past trauma or hardships. Each one of these individuals chose not to dwell on it, but persevered and maintained a sense of humor, in spite of whatever difficulty was present.

As we thought about the values and grace of those we interviewed, we became aware of the many important facets shaping their lives. For example, we were impressed by the fact that food was such a central theme in each person's life. It represented family traditions, forms of celebration, and just plain comfort when made by relatives or friends as a labor of love. Many folks reminisced about homemade cooking from scratch and lamented that our family lives today are so demanding that we can't take the time to "eat from the land," dine in a relaxed fashion, and enjoy nice table settings, tasty food, and conversation.

Our fast-paced society prevents us from sharing our legacy with others—stories, poems, and words of advice—which others will benefit from as a result of our experience. We are leaving our "material" wills to our children, but we are neglecting to write down our advice on things we have valued. It is our sincere hope that the stories in this book will encourage our readers to record their own stories. Such a legacy is one of the most precious gifts you can leave to your children, nieces, nephews, grandchildren, and great-grandchildren. It will provide a context for their lives and be a source of lasting joy. Additionally, the practical information you provide can be of benefit in their own lives.

We ourselves have learned to live more purposeful lives as a result of this endeavor. For the past several months, I have been thinking about the grandmother I would love to be one day. I remember walking on a beach last summer memorizing how to build unusual sandcastles to eventually make with my grandkids. I have already chosen a spot in the yard where I will teach them how to grow beautiful flowers. And, in one room of my home, I have saved a special corner for all the books I hope to read to them. I even have a box of dress-up clothes ready for them to enjoy as they explore their creative selves near a piano I hope to play while they dance and improvise. I know the kind of parent I was, and I want to share things with my kids that I have learned when they too someday become parents.

As we reflected on the lives of the men and women we interviewed, we tried to identify some essential guiding beliefs that would be of particular relevance in our own lives. Hence, each vignette begins with a reflection of our own, and the end of the book will provide an opportunity for our readers to record their own legacies. It is our hope that each reader, depending on his or her own experiences and needs, will be touched by some particular aspect of the stories that are shared here and will benefit and be affected in a way that enriches their understanding and is personally meaningful.

CONTENTS

LISTEN TO THE WISEST OF ALL

PROFILES

RUTH YOUNGERMAN

An exuberant, dignified, meticulously groomed ninety-three-year-old woman of small stature greeted us at the door of her home as though we were long-lost friends. We fell easily into conversation. Philosophical remarks permeated our discussion along with phrases, sayings, and good old words of advice from parents, family and friends she adored. Without hesitation, Ruth Youngerman began sharing her favorite words of wisdom as we sat down for the first time in her living room: "If you want something, ask yourself if you need it." "Life is better if you pace yourself." "It's not what you say, it's what you do." The most poignant quotation for Kim and me was when Ruth looked up at us and said, "No two families are ever the same. You don't understand a man until you know his memories."

Another important concept Ruth values is simplicity: "Simplicity brings you closer to reality. Our needs and wants are miles apart." The more you have, the more you have to take care of." This vibrant woman attributes her long life to good genes, a favorable environment, enjoying nature, healthy eating, and much luck. She feels lucky to have played golf and tennis until she was eighty years old; soon after, Ruth began practicing tai chi. Ruth also loved being in her backyard as much as possible. Her Mother's Day gift every other year from her husband was a new lawn mower. After cutting her grass, Ruth loved feeling the blades of grass under her feet—a simple pleasure she relished.

Ruth's birthplace was in Illinois where small farming communities surrounded her. She believes that "people who are brought up on farms and surrounded by nature are more fulfilled than people who live in cities surrounded by concrete." Ruth is thankful that she was brought up in a small community, which was a peaceful setting where she could contemplate God and feel close to nature. Urban folks are "too tight and compact with their cold subways and neighbors who don't know one another and have too many distractions."

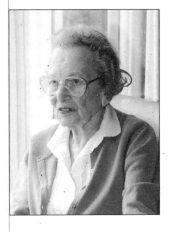

AGE: 93
"Accept the fact that in each decade of your life you will think differently."

Authors' Reflection:
"It's important to make children work so they appreciate things and don't develop a sense of entitlement."

1

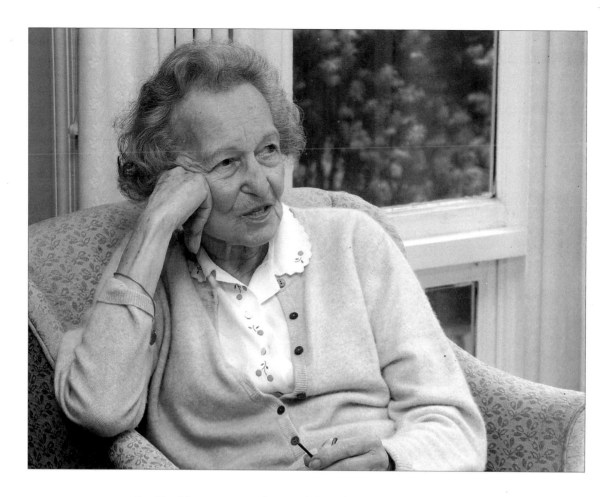

In Ruth's opinion, the world today is competitive and uncooperative. Reality is now based on motion pictures and television rather than direct experiences with others. She remembers that in the early days people got pleasure out of helping each other. Ruth feels that now everyone is trying to get to the top of the ladder at the expense of others. Her parents instilled in her the value of giving rather than receiving. Ruth particularly enjoyed reminiscing about the way her father did business in the "old days." Farmers would come into his dry-goods store complaining that the shoes he had sold them weren't any good. Although Ruth's father knew that the shoes were three years old, he didn't want to shame his customers and always gave them new shoes. In more profitable years, her father would give the extra money to employees. He never kept it for himself. Ruth's father also bought property on which to build houses for his employees. That was his pleasure, according to Ruth. He always practiced the credo that "anonymous giving is the best."

Looking back, Ruth remembers wanting different things for herself during each decade of her life. During one decade, she and her contemporaries valued physical beauty. In another decade, they strove for achievement. Ruth remembers wondering whether she was living the life she intended, and whether she would someday have any regrets about her decisions. Her advice to us and to others was to accept disappointments, ambivalences, and past decisions, knowing that at the time one does the best one can. To look back with regret would be a grave mistake.

As Ruth looked outside her window, she commented on the mature trees in her yard and how massive the vegetation had gotten over the years. It reminded her of children who grow up too quickly in our society. Ruth said, "Kids are too mature these days. They don't have things and events to look forward to as we did. They travel to Europe and other places even before high school, and all are given the luxury of material consumption before they are old enough to appreciate it. If children don't have something, they get it. We didn't have that sense of entitlement when we were younger. We wrote in diaries, danced, played outside, and were disciplined strongly. No child would ever think about throwing something on the ground. We respected other people and their property. I think discipline is a very helpful and happy thing to have."

As we chatted, Ruth excused herself and several minutes later came back with a tea cart, dainty china cups, napkins with a floral print, and tea cookies. To many contemporary women, serving afternoon tea is an act from a bygone era. To Kim and me it was a pure delight, an example of "going the

extra mile," and something we greatly appreciated. It made us want to serve more graciously and more often in our own homes. Perhaps friends might pause a moment in their hectic lives to savor conversation with us, being treated to place settings that included more than a simple coffee mug.

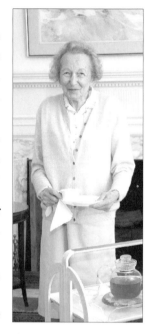

As we sipped tea, Ruth told us about her husband and her children. Her husband, William, had been a prominent physician. Ruth appreciated his philosophy of marriage: "Each partner should give 125%." Ruth added that "couples now expect too much of each other." Ruth has been a widow for over thirty years. She and her husband had three children, two boys and a girl. One memory Ruth shared as we were talking was how she enjoyed teaching her children five new vocabulary words from the *Readers Digest* each morning at breakfast. Since Ruth remembers being corrected a lot as a child, she made a point of complimenting her children. "One never knows what your child experiences. I would rather have an 'over-secure child.' That is very important. It is very hard to build yourself up if you have that 'armored coat' on."

When asked to comment on the technological advances in our society, Ruth vehemently responded that she always wants to hear from her children by telephone and not through e-mail. "That's when you know how your children are really feeling emotionally. Your children can talk beautifully on the telephone, yet there is something you get from the tone in their voice." When asked about organized religion, she responded that rituals and holiday celebrations have always been more important to her than dogma.

Ruth's basic but all encompassing philosophy has been "to always follow the Golden Rule."

Presently, Ruth enjoys public television and radio, "Sunday Morning" with Charles Osgood, British comedies, and "Everybody Loves Raymond." She claims that she doesn't have a lot of time to watch TV. Before Ruth gets out of bed in the morning, she does a few exercises. After she has breakfast and gets dressed, she does her paperwork, including handling her own finances. Some days Ruth picks up some friends who can't drive anymore and goes out to eat or shopping. For over fifty years, Ruth has belonged to a play-reading club in which the members read a short play out loud. "We start in September and end in May. Over the summer we have a committee that chooses the plays for the upcoming year." She is still active in the Art Club. Founded in 1870, it is actually about the art of conversation, with members presenting different subjects to the group. Having a little hot toddy around 5:30 p.m. is still a ritual for Ruth at the end of each day.

Ruth continued chatting, sitting in her comfortable chair surrounded by novels, photography books, and newspaper clippings. She picked up an Anne Geddes book with pictures of children's faces, which made her laugh spontaneously. She leaned back and confided, "Children are the only ones I really trust. Their laughter is a gift from heaven." Kiddingly, Ruth told us that a couple of months ago she realized that she wasn't going to live forever. She thinks it will take her a while to get rid of things in her house before she moves to a retirement village. She looked around her house and commented that years ago children loved getting things of sentimental value from their parents. "Life is different now. All the kids want to do is to travel and see things. They don't enjoy just staying home anymore."

Ruth still misses the many friends she has survived in her ninety-three years. "I wish there were a group of seniors close to my age that got together as a formal support group for one another." Ruth said that she enjoyed hearing

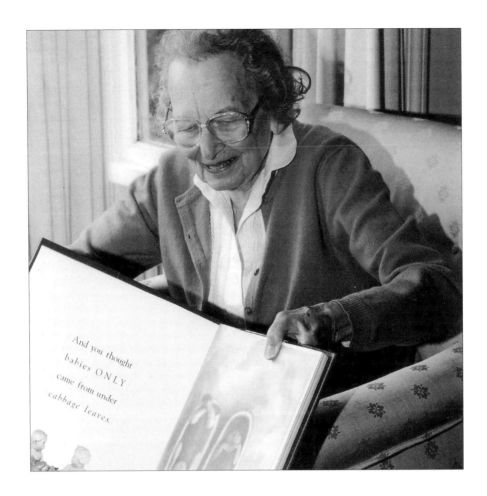

about things from a female and male perspective. "Friendship is flavored by companionship and conversation. I used to admire friends who played a good game of golf. Now that I am older I admire people who have done a lot of worthwhile things in their lives." As Ruth continued to contemplate her life and the different types of people she has met, she remarked that she has received the most pleasure from simple people rather than from the affluent people whom she periodically encountered. As we were leaving Ruth's home one day, we noticed two passages prominently displayed on her refrigerator. As we walked a few steps to read them, Ruth commented to us that these were her favorite sayings: "Accept the unacceptable" and "There are no great men, only great challenges which ordinary men are forced by necessity to meet."

MARY AVANT

At four years of age, Mary Avant witnessed her three-year-old sister, Georgia, burn to death in a house fire. After experiencing this tragedy at such a young age, Mary felt a need for caution and vigilance and developed her life-long philosophy, which she expressed in one sentence: "Think before you leap." At ninety-seven, Mary still practices this credo, as when, for example, she decided not to use a credit card to buy something she realized she really didn't need. As Mary shared her story with us, we were struck by the discipline and perseverance that have marked her life.

Of all the people we interviewed Mary had the heartiest laugh, and ironically, the hardest life. She always dressed in matching pantsuits and cute necklaces, earrings, and bracelets. We asked Mary why she got dressed up even when she stayed at home, and she replied, "If you have jewelry, wear it even if you can't go out. It makes a person feel better. It also makes me feel better when I wake up, get dressed, and know that there are leftovers in the fridge." Mary, who lives with her daughter and grandson, told us that she wants to do as much for herself as she can for as long as she can, but appreciates the help given to her by family and friends. She described with great delight a homemade coconut pie—her favorite—which her daughter had brought her. She still is able to travel; recently she visited her sister in Mississippi, where she enjoyed a bit of gambling. With characteristic discipline, Mary set a $50 per day limit for herself and did not exceed it.

The daughter of sharecroppers in Mississippi, Mary vividly recalled her early life in the cotton fields. She spoke of picking the cotton, taking it to be baled, and watching her parents getting paid by the "white folk." As Mary described this experience, she looked down at her fingers, the skin of which was rough and cracked from years of hard work. She reminisced about how the children in her family, as young as ten years, picked the cotton and took it to the gin to have the seeds removed and to be weighed.

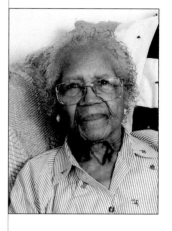

AGE: 97
"Think before you leap."

Authors' Reflection:
"There is great value in making a well thought-out decision before you act."

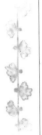

Mary remembered that the "sack weight," or the weight for which they were paid, often was quite a bit less than what they had carried to the gin. After the seed was taken out at the gin, the workers would bale the cotton. It took about fifteen or sixteen sacks of cotton to get a bale, which averaged 490 pounds net weight. Mary loved describing the cotton fields and the cotton plants. During one of our interviews, she showed us some cottonseed that friends had brought back from Mississippi. "Cottonseed is planted just like a flower." The plant grows and flowers, and she told us that each flower made a boll. When the boll opened, the cotton inside was "pure white." Then it was picked. Mary looked up at us proudly and said, "This is what your clothes are made of."

Mary described her home of origin in Mississippi as a "shotgun house." When you entered the front door you could look right through to the back door. It had three bedrooms, a kitchen, and a smokehouse. The smokehouse was where they put their pork and anything else that was "killed." She described the different parts of the pig, where different kinds of meat came from, including the "side, where you got the bacon," and, with a bit of a grimace, the chitlins. Meat was washed and salted in the spring. Her parents then hung the meat up in the smokehouse and smoked it for hours. Certain wood chips were used to give the right flavor to the meat. All of Mary's family members ate this food for the entire year. To this day Mary says that she doesn't care for ham because of that process. "I raised my hams and I had enough of that!"

When asked if her mother taught her to cook, she quickly responded that there was no teaching. "I just watched my Mama." Mary's Dad built a little platform around the stove for her to stand on and be able to reach everything. She told us an amusing story about her attempt to make a cake after she had watched her mother. She described how her mother put the eggs,

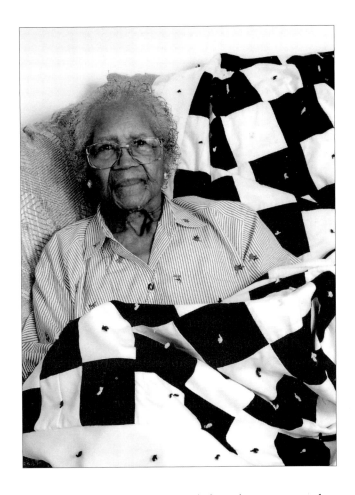

sugar, and flour in the bowl. Giggling, Mary said that she put everything in her "experimental" cake, but forgot to add the flour. Her cake boiled over and burned up. Undaunted, she resolved to watch her mother bake again, and this time she watched more closely. She made the next cake with buttermilk but didn't put any soda in it. Another mess appeared in her oven. She then blurted out, "I am going to make this cake and I will keep going until it comes out right"—and she did.

Although Mary shared the responsibility of cooking for her large family, including eight brothers and sisters, she was also determined to learn to sew and quilt. When her mother would go to the cotton field and leave Mary at

the house to care for the other children, she would take little pieces of material, roll them together, and use the scraps for quilting. Mary would put the babies in the family to sleep and get out her mother's sewing machine. She would hide the quilt she was making because she wanted to surprise her mother. When Mary presented the finished quilt, her mother was amazed. She asked Mary where the quilt had come from, and Mary proudly said, "I made it." Unfortunately, one day Mary stuck a machine needle through her finger. (She showed Kim and me a scar on her finger where the sewing-machine needle had gone straight through.) She never told her mother about it because she knew she wouldn't let her continue to use the sewing machine. Mary went on to make clothes for herself and her siblings. Jokingly, she said that she always made the dresses for her sisters exactly alike so no one would feel superior. Mary not only made clothes for her family but also washed them by hand. Later, she sewed for other kids who, as Mary put it, "didn't have a Mama." Gradually, people from neighboring towns heard about her skill and would bring clothes for her to alter. As time went on, they would not only come to Mary for her sewing, but also bring their kids to the house so she could comb and fix their hair. One day a little girl who was very dirty appeared on her doorstep. She proceeded to wrap this girl in a towel, wash her clothes by hand, and hang them out to dry. Mary was only twelve years old at the time, and she was proud to see this little girl so clean and neat.

Mary told us that there wasn't much time for good, clean fun in her day. She tried to enjoy herself, though, and thought of games to entertain herself and her friends. Mary enjoyed telling us a story about what happened to her at the age of nine. She was in her house cleaning so that she could go outside and play, but when she got outside none of her friends were there. With nothing better to do, she climbed up on an old woodpile and challenged herself to say the alphabet backward. As she was telling this story, Mary sat up quite erectly and, without pausing for a second, recited the entire alphabet backward! Kim and I were completely astonished at this ninety-seven-year-old woman who had just easily demonstrated a verbal feat we knew would befuddle us.

Another childhood memory involved the cows that Mary's family raised. Being strong willed, she got up on one of the cows and tried to ride it for fun. The cow would get close to the trees and try to brush her off, but she never fell off her "horse." In those days, Mary befriended a group of boys. She considered herself to be a tomboy and wanted to do everything the boys did. A boy would climb a pecan tree on a Sunday and knock down the nuts with his fishing pole. The next Sunday would be her turn. She would climb the tree and shake the limbs in hopes that lots of pecans would fall. She giggled as she was telling this story because she said she could never come down from the tree alone – she always needed the boys to help her.

Married at only fourteen, Mary made sure that we understood that she wasn't pregnant at the time. She married one of the neighbor boys. They were married for fifty-eight years and he died at the age of seventy-two. Together they had eight children, four boys and four girls. Sadly, Mary's oldest daughter died at the age of sixteen. Mary confided that as the years went by, the weight of her sadness slowly lifted. She has also survived two sons. When we asked Mary if she was in love at the time she married, she replied that she wasn't sure. Unfortunately, her husband drank excessively. She said that her husband drank "white lightning" and would forget their conversations. This experience completely turned her against marriage. When asked what makes a good marriage, Mary retorted, "I don't know because I didn't have one!"

Until very recently, quilting was Mary's greatest passion in life. She made many beautiful quilts and even won prizes at quilt shows. Now she enjoys watching television during the day, especially soap operas. Although she

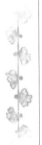

doesn't bake very much any more, she doesn't like to buy cake mixes. "I would rather make it from scratch." Talking on the phone to family members and friends is one of the highlights of Mary's day. She also rides her exercise bicycle, which stands in her hallway. Pointing to her leg, she said, "When I get this straightened out, I ride my bicycle for exercise. I just keep on pushin'. I make sure that my daughter who is turning seventy years of age isn't allowed to use the word *old.*" Mary tells her not to think old, but to think young. At night Mary enjoys watching the news. She likes to go to bed and watch TV until she falls asleep.

When questioned about disciplining children, Mary strongly felt that kids need spankings. In her day, parents would have the right to spank other people's misbehaving children. "These days you better not hit a kid. This is some of what is wrong with the world. Another thing that is wrong with the world is that young women are going around naked. They show their rumps and their breasts. What do these women expect? If these girls don't have respect for themselves, why do they think anyone would?" Mary feels that kids don't work hard enough. "When I was young, I got out there and sweated and worked for something. That's how I got things. I also feel like people don't put enough effort into raising their kids. Kids are so hateful sometimes that you are afraid of letting them in your house."

Looking back on her life, Mary is glad she left Mississippi and moved to Illinois. Initially, she came to Illinois to visit some friends, but she soon realized that her life would be better if she moved permanently. Reflecting on her life in Mississippi, she explained that they had to have wood to heat their houses in the winter and in Illinois she could conveniently push a button. There were no furnaces where she had lived. It was hard to leave family and friends behind, but Mary and her family persevered, made new friends, and created a new life for themselves.

When Mary was asked to what she attributed her longevity, she thought for a long time. Finally, she told us that she owed her long life to having had a lot of sympathy for people when she was growing up. She said that if she had a little more than the other person, she wanted to "take that person along with me. I always loved lending a helping hand to others. Many people get lots of things in their lifetime and then tromp all over you. I always had sympathy for people who looked like they had less than me. I think God has given me a long life because of this."

When asked if she could share her thoughts on how this generation of families could live a better life, Mary emphatically stated: "Hard work is important, tell the truth always, and don't let your fingers stick to any-thing—that is stealing."

ORVAL & MAE TRIMBLE

"There is nothing better than a good waltz or cha-cha," reminisced 102-year-old Orval. As we sat down at the kitchen table listening to stories about their ballroom-dancing days, ninety-five-year-old Mae mentioned that they retired from dancing when Orval celebrated his 100th birthday. However, music has always been and still is a big part of their lives individually and as a couple. Orval began playing the fiddle in elementary school. He was determined to learn to play well, and he practiced every day. Orval told us that one day when "I got to sawin' on my fiddle," his folks told him he had better go in the back room. Orval laughed as he told this story, but he said he never gave up and became quite good. As an adult he played for square dances at all the surrounding country towns. His first wife, Belle, was a great square dancer and she also played the banjo. He and his wife would often play at hootenannies, where different bands would perform thirty-minute gigs while people danced the night away. "The countryside is a great place for those types of things," he recalled with pleasure. After Orval married his second wife, Mae, they would follow his son's band and dance to the sounds of big band music. That's when they realized that they needed ballroom-dancing lessons.

Orval had twin brothers, who were ten years younger, and one sister, but he is the only one still living. He showed us an old community-band picture of him and his brothers in which he is proudly wearing a bow tie. That bow tie became his trademark at an early age and it continues to be to this day. We laughed as we noticed a pin on the table that read, "I have survived damn near everything!" This pin was given to Orval at his 100th birthday party, which their dance instructor attended.

During his working life, corn husking was Orval's favorite activity. He was in many local and county competitions and often took first place. He obviously loved talking about the process, as well as about all the cattle he had

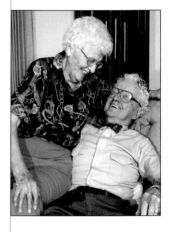

AGE: 95 & 102
"Sometimes we wake up in the morning and we are still holding hands."

Authors' Reflection:
"Hard work is the key to a healthy mind and life."

15

raised. Reflecting on his family's years of farming, Orval commented on the Great Depression. He remembers the banks closing and the fact that it would cost them more to haul the pigs to market than they would earn selling them. Fortunately, if you lived on a farm, you got most of your good food living off the land. He farmed in his community of birth until the river "bottomed out" in 1929. After that he found work farther north and drove two days and most of one night to reach his job. He recalled that there wasn't a light on the road. "I drove through the country and was out there with six head of horses. Two teams coming up the road and all I could see was a lantern once in a while or a home with a kerosene light on in the house." As Orval talked about this period, he picked up the "pin" on the table as a testament to his surviving those rough times.

Although Orval quit school after eighth grade to farm, he talked about some of his school memories and the fact that he was so proud of learning compound interest. He loved figuring in his head, and he believed that he could do it more quickly than if he had used a calculator. "Technology can make a person lazy. Doing the math in your head keeps you sharp and alive," he declared. He plowed the entire farm with six horses—using two teams, with a set of three in front and three in back. He had a board on the plow, and he would stand up on that board with two sets of lines.

When Orval was a young boy, he watched his grandfather raising bees and harvesting honey in the wintertime. Although Orval didn't work with the bees himself, he would help by cleaning the beehives for hours at a time. The bees didn't bother his grandpa, according to Orval, "because he didn't pay attention to them." However, his grandpa would carry a smoker with him, and if there were too many bees, he would hit the smoker and they would drift away. Orval clearly loved sharing that memory.

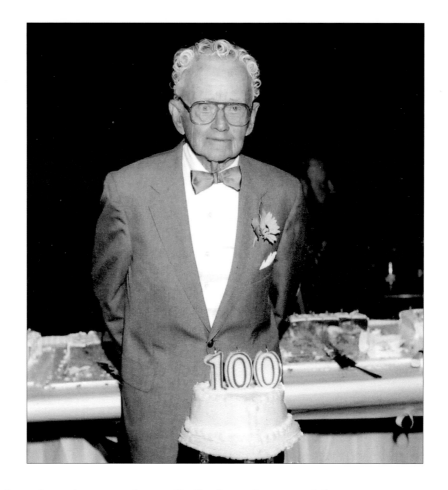

Orval was happily married to Belle for forty-five years. They met at a pie supper. In those days women would bake pies, and the men bid on the pies. As fate would have it, Orval bid on Belle's pie. Once the bidding was over, the men would sit with the women and eat a piece of pie together. That was the beginning of Orval and Belle's relationship. He loved her cooking, and he said that she was a good mother and the best square dancer around. They had three children, two boys and one girl. When Belle got sick, Mae was her nurse in the hospital, and after Belle passed away, Orval and Mae began dating. They just celebrated thirty-five years of marriage.

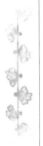

As Mae began telling us about her childhood growing up in Kentucky, we moved to the living room to sit on the sofa. Orval and Mae were quite attentive to one another during these conversations, and we noticed the constant glances and touches between them. Mae was born in a two-story log cabin. There were no amenities in the house; they had an outhouse but no store-bought toilet paper. She loved her mother's cooking, especially her biscuits. Her mother made biscuits three times a day and cornbread once a day.

Mae spent a good deal of time talking about her parents' working in the tobacco patch and she described the whole process, including when the tobacco got really tall and the plants were thickly infested with worms. She told us that she would scream at the sight of the worms, and she giggled as she recalled that memory. Her father would grab the worms and tear their heads off. He would then take a special knife and cut the plants. Afterward, he would put several plants on a stick and hang the stick in the barn until they dried. He would take the tobacco plants off the sticks and bring them into the house. At this point in the story, Mae laughed heartily as she recalled her mother's reaction to the mess this made on her floors. Her father would then start stripping the leaves from the tobacco. The bud leaves were the choice ones, and Mae explained that cigar coverings were made from these. "These were the better leaves as dad used the bottom leaves for cigarettes." After this process was completed, Mae's dad would load a big wagon and drive to the closest town. The tobacco was shipped by train to Louisville, and her dad would follow on the train to sell it.

Another of Mae's fond memories was sitting on the porch swing with her grandma and grandpa as they watched passersby on the road. She said, "They would each smoke a pipe after dinner. Grandpa had a fancy curved pipe, and my grandma's pipe was smooth and much smaller." During this time, Mae would sit on her grandpa's lap and braid his long white beard over and over.

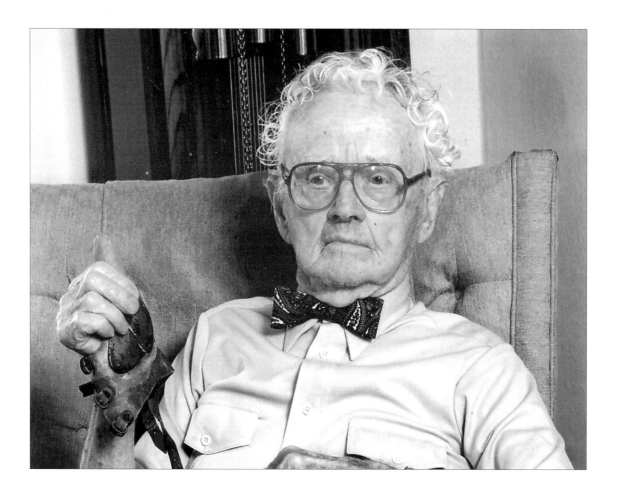

We were curious about what a typical day consisted of for Orval and Mae. Arising between 5:30 and 6:00 a.m., they have a small breakfast of cereal and orange juice. Orval doesn't like orange juice, but Mae forces him to drink it. Mae pointed out that years ago when they were farming they had eggs, bacon, and a "whole big meal" for breakfast. After breakfast, Mae washes the dishes and makes the bed. Then she feeds the cats. Proudly, Mae exclaimed, "Then my housework is done. Sometimes I do bake pies in the afternoon." When asked what Orval's favorite pie was, he quickly responded pumpkin. Mae mentioned that Orval likes her scalloped pine-apple casserole, too. After lunch, they take a one-hour nap. On certain days

Mae drives herself to the beauty shop. In the evening they sit and talk, as they find nothing on television that really interests them any more. Because Orval's eyes are failing, Mae reads to him. Sometimes they listen to big band music in the evening as well.

Each spring, even at 102 and 95 years of age, they excitedly look forward to mowing the lawn with their twin lawn mowers. Their faces lit up when they described the smell of the freshly cut grass. They laughed as they described their "female and male" mowers that they love to use for two or three hours at a time. This spring they plan to move Mae's dad's peony bush near the house so they can see it and also have it close to Orval's father's peony bush. This peony bush is one of the "old-fashioned short ones," according to Mae, and its beautiful red blossoms appear early in the spring when Orval and Mae long for bursts of nature to come forth. The couple enjoys their gardening activities, and they still reminisce about Orval's getting on his hands and knees to dig his potatoes out of the garden.

We couldn't wait to ask Orval and Mae to what they attributed their longevity. They both answered loudly in unison—"hard work." Orval added that he has weighed 126 pounds all his adult life. It was clear that these two special people still remained filled with the joy of living. They also offered some clear-cut advice: "Kids have to be disciplined regardless of how parents choose to do it," and "Be completely honest with one another in a marriage."

During the last ten minutes of our conversation, although it was hard for us to broach this sensitive subject, we asked them if they were afraid of death. Mae said, "I dread it because we are so happy together that I just hate to part." Orval's answer was, "Whatever happens, happens." At that moment, Orval grabbed Mae's hand and said, "Sometimes we wake up in the morning and we are still holding hands."

JOE HAMBURG

AMERICA IS A WONDERFUL PLACE

"*Baruch haShem Yom Yom.*" This Hebrew expression means, "Thank you dear God for allowing us to be together again today." Ninety-three-year-old Joseph Hamburg and his longtime friends recite these words when they gather at a different restaurant each week as the "Thursday Lunch Bunch" or the "Old Farts" as Joe loves to say. Joe looks forward to this weekly lunch date. "It's a good mixture of men with different interests. Everyone has something to share. Some men are less talkative, others are a little more rambunctious and say things to challenge us. We always talk about current events and also matters that are dear to our hearts."

As we sat in his living room, Joe shared stories with us about the people he cherished—his wife, his family, and close friends. "My wife was, and still is, my best friend. Merle and I weathered being apart during the war, loved raising our son, and now are thankful that we can see our grandson and his children." He and his wife worked together at the family-owned dry-cleaning business and together enjoyed the camaraderie of other business owners. Joe went on to sing Merle's praises: "She was an excellent cook and baker and a very good mother. I loved her casseroles, her cakes, her brownies, croissants, and coffee cakes. I always complimented her, and she knew that I meant it. She knew that I valued this labor of love very much. Merle never followed a recipe. She learned her cooking skills as a young bride in Europe would have learned. Most of what Merle learned was from her mother. Merle was proud that she learned how to make gefilte fish and matzo ball soup, 'Jewish delicacies' in my opinion. We have had a fun-filled and memorable marriage."

We asked Joe his advice on what makes a good marriage. "You have to be sure that you truly love the person you are marrying. When a person takes his or her wedding vows, they make a lifelong commitment to love, honor, and cherish, as they say. I think married couples need to be completely faithful,

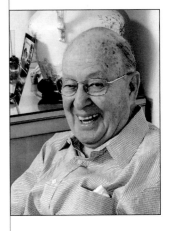

AGE: 93
"Be a good citizen of the world. It all comes back to you."

Authors' Reflection:
"To be born into a good family is a lucky gift, but developing a true friendship is an immeasurable and even greater gift."

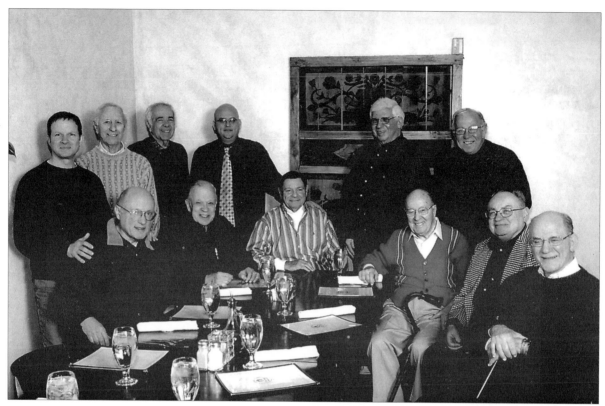

"Thursday Lunch Bunch"

loving, understanding, tolerant, and not demanding of one another. Couples, in my opinion, need to have pretty much the same degree of intelligence, education, and common sense. You need to like some things in common. For example, my wife and I both loved the arts. We were frequent visitors at the Krannert Center for the Performing Arts in Urbana, Illinois, which is actually modeled after New York's Lincoln Center."

We continued our discussion about friends. "I think friends are a very important part of a person's life. You know that saying, 'You can't choose your family, but you can choose your friends.' We were fortunate to make a lot of good friends. Our dear friends are a treasure. We have friends we have known for fifty or more years." Joe shared a parody of the song "Thanks for the Memories" that he wrote and tearfully sang in honor of his close friend, Arthur, whom he has known for sixty-six years. Joe emphasized to us that friendships are well worth the time and commitment they require because they enhance one's life so much.

As we were talking to Joe, we noticed medals on the wall including the Purple Heart. He responded with humility when we pointed them out, but we could sense that he was proud of his accomplishments. He told us that he didn't like to focus on negative things but was willing to chat a little about his feelings regarding war. "War is hell," Joe stated vehemently. "You don't know from one day to the next if you are going to be alive." Joe entered the war at twenty-nine. Soon after being deployed, he realized how many things in his life he had taken for granted. He was married almost five years when he had to go into the army. His wife was pregnant, and the baby was born after he finished basic training. Unfortunately, he had to wait until he got his first leave to see his son at four-and-a-half months of age. Immediately after seeing his son, Joe received orders to be shipped overseas. He was assigned to the Second Infantry Division and served in Normandy, France. In the early stages of his assignment, he saw a big air armada that flew over the beaches at Normandy. It was the largest aerial bombing that had ever taken place in the history of the United States. Soon after, Joe and his army companions saw smoke bombs come down, and they knew that this was the bombing of St. Lô, which was the turning point of the war. That was when General Patton and his army started to battle their way through France. Joe witnessed this in July of 1944, and he did not return home until December of 1945.

Since Joe's dry-cleaning business allowed him to observe clothing styles over the years, we asked him his opinion of contemporary dress. "Most people in today's society want to be more casual. No one wants to get dressed

up. Even in very high corporate positions, men are wearing jackets and leaving out ties. On Fridays some companies are completely casual and men wear a sweater or sport shirt." He commented on the cyclical nature of dress, even beginning with the days of Henry VIII and Queen Elizabeth I. "In those days the necklines were all low. Then there were times when the ladies wore dresses with high necklines and long sleeves." As time progressed, he remembered more changes in dress. Although Joe doesn't describe himself as being old-fashioned, he disapproves of immodest clothes. He doesn't feel it is ladylike to expose so much skin, such as bare midriffs and so much cleavage. With a nostalgic tone in his voice, Joe remembered when women routinely wore dresses and heels, and on special occasions, added hats and gloves. "That was class," Joe exclaimed. "Today I know that the young people are very bright, but I am disappointed when I see kids dressing in a ragged fashion or having hair that looks unclean." Joe feels it shows lack of pride and, possibly, demonstrates low self-esteem.

The many family photographs we saw on Joe's apartment walls aroused our curiosity about his background. He vividly remembered the stories of his ancestors. "My parents decided in their thirties to emigrate to the United States. They were living in a small town in western Russia close to the Lithuanian border with their four children when they made this decision to emigrate." Joe gives them a lot of credit for leaving their homes and their countries and traveling 3,000 miles to a strange land at the turn of the century. They had no relatives in the United States, and they couldn't speak a word of English. Joe's father came over first with his oldest son and found work as a carpenter and skilled cabinetmaker. The son worked as an assistant to a tailor. He saved for two years and then sent for the rest of the family, which included Joe's mother, two more sons, and a daughter. Joe's father met them at Ellis Island, the port of entry in New York City where so many new immigrants began their lives in this country. Joe talked about people coming to America from Poland, Ireland, Italy, Germany, Czechoslovakia, and the whole Baltic region.

In their new country, the family missed the small-town atmosphere in Russia where everyone knew one another and each person's Yiddish name. Joe's parents frequently talked about their homeland and how their house was a meeting place for all of their cronies. Joe always pictured the type of place his parents must have had and compared it to the setting of *Fiddler on the Roof.* Of course, his parents were never able to return because of pogroms—massacres of "undesirable" people back in Russia. Joe's mother was overwhelmed by the size of New York City. "She told my father right away, 'I do not like the big city. I want to live in a little *shtetl* [a small town].'" Joe said that his father saw the handwriting on the wall, and he wasn't going to try to change her mind. So his father enlisted the help of the Hebrew Immigrant Aid Society. This organization was helpful in finding the right homes for new immigrants who were coming over at that time from Poland, Ireland, Italy, Germany, and other places. The Society found a prominent family to sponsor Joe's parents, and that was how the Hamburgs came to live in the Midwest. After settling in the United States, they had three more children.

Joe felt strongly that this wave of immigration was a great benefit for people with a strong work ethic, declaring, "America is a wonderful place. All of the different immigrants came over starting in the middle part of the nineteenth century and melded together to make this great country like it is today. Immigrants from many parts of the world, such as the Mexicans, Asians, Jews, and other ethnic groups have all assimilated and worked hard to elevate their position in America."

After sharing so many experiences with us, Joe emphasized what a good feeling it was for him to reminisce about his life. Joe talked about his early

years. He described how his mother had her hands full with young children and a husband who was extremely busy earning a living. Joe's parents went into the grocery business, and since they were so busy night and day, they didn't have a lot of time to discipline the children. Joe told us that they were good children and good students. He and his siblings did a lot of mentoring work with students who were having difficulty in class. For fun Joe and his siblings would go to the local theatre, which showed silent movies. The kids loved their Monday night tradition of going to movies, delighting in Westerns or mystery stories. During this era of silent movies, the piano player sat near the screen right down in front of the theatre. He would play exceedingly fast for a horse race, and then change to a melancholy mood for a sad story. After sound was introduced, the wonderful musicals of the forties were produced and that was a big thrill.

"As children," he said, "we used to be excited about football games. I never had enough money to be able to buy a ticket and go watch the games, but I used to go and sit outside the stadium with a group of kids. There was no radio as a means of communication. When a team scored a touchdown, a cannon would be shot off. After the shell exploded several hundred feet in the air, a parachute would come out and it would have the colors of the school that scored the touchdown. As the parachute floated downward, the kids would hurry to try to get one as a souvenir."

Reflecting on his life, Joe stated, "I had and presently have a great appreciation for living. I am sad that my wife can't be with me in this retirement village. She needs to be in a nursing home because of the kind of care that she gets. But I talk to her several times a day and see her whenever I can. However, I never like to dwell on sad things. I like to write musical parodies that honor all the special people in my life and all the memories that I have. I don't fear death. When I was younger I feared it much more. I do

Thanks for the Memories

Thanks for the memories,
Of six years, plus three score
We hope there're many more
The friendship of our families,
Will last forevermore—
How lucky we are

Thanks for the memories,
When married life was new
Our friendship grew and grew,
Our families expanded,
You had many—
We had few—
We've surely been blessed

Our life has been great, I'm confessing,
Enrichment by friends, what a blessing
The joy of all this I'm expressing—
We had a ball, and that's not all

I feel there's much more in store—
We'll go on as we are and earn our "just
reward"
Which Providence will grant us—
As we say, "Thank you dear Lord,"
And I thank you so much—yes—
I thank you so much!

Many more happy birthdays, Arthur!

06/05

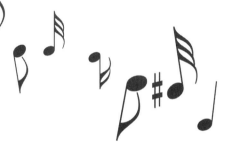

A parody written by Joe Hamburg

want to continue living because I am interested in seeing how the world is going to be with all of the great technology we have. I love starting my day each morning with 'CNN' and 'The View.' Every week I attend a Rotary meeting. I have always been proud to be a Rotarian. I never miss watching 'Oprah' and 'Larry King Live.' I love to hear stimulating conversation with people who are interesting and have common sense. Of course, I always have to watch 'The Price Is Right' and 'Wheel of Fortune'—that is a long-standing tradition of mine.

"I also love to draw, which has been an avocation of mine for many years. I have done faces of some members of our family. My newest great-grand-

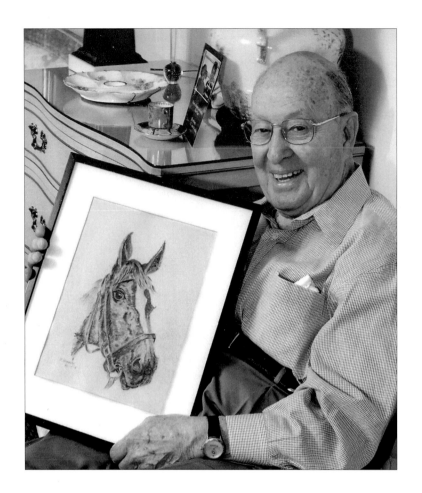

daughter is little Goldie. My next goal is to complete a drawing of her. I love listening to my grandson share stories about his parenting of his own children. Grandparents are important. My grandson is very lucky, as he has grandparents on both sides of the family. I wasn't able to enjoy the company of a grandparent, and I am sad about that."

We asked Joe for his advice and views on a healthy and fulfilling life. After pondering this question for a while, he stressed how important it was to be a good person: to have good morals and to be kind, understanding, helpful, charitable, and also to have an appreciation for the arts. "Be a good person, a good husband or wife, and good grandparent. Be a good citizen of the world. It all comes back to you."

LOUISE FOGELSANGER

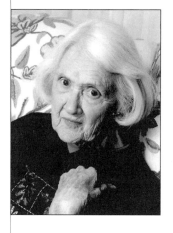

AGE: 92
"Be considerate,
look at things as
a whole, practice
tolerance."

"Happy" greeted us at the back door. Happy is the beloved dog owned by Virginia Louise Fogelsanger, a charming ninety-two-year-old woman whom we had the good fortune to interview. Happy immediately demanded our attention, which clearly was fine with Louise. Our warm response to her dog obviously gave her a great deal of pride and pleasure—a feeling that all pet owners know so well. Even before we formally introduced ourselves, Louise told us that we must be nice people because her dog instantly approved of us.

Louise is a dignified, white-haired woman with a slight southern accent. Her clothes were lovely and obviously new. While we stroked the top of Happy's head, we told Louise lightheartedly that she didn't need to get dressed up for our interview. She mentioned that she had been a size 16, but as a result of losing weight after a bad fall, she was now a size 10 and the owner of many fashionable new clothes. We later realized that this response embodied the essence of Louise's personality—always reframing things in a positive way. We eventually learned that she had acquired this wonderful trait from her "hero," her father.

Louise loved talking about her dad. One could feel the deep respect she had for him. He ran a country dry-goods store when she was growing up, and customers would come into the store to buy things, visit, and share some gossip. As a matter of principle, her father would never repeat anything said to him in confidence, even to Louise's mother. He would give Louise a little kick under the table as her mother prodded him for information, and Louise would giggle. Her mother knew that all the children favored their father over her. "I know you all like your dad better, but I picked him," she would say with a grin. During the Depression, Louise's father let people have credit even though her family didn't have much themselves. Her concerned mother would question this and ask, "Why do you keep letting these

Authors' Reflection:
"If you really feel
the music, you won't
notice a few sour
notes."

29

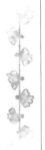

people have food?" He would answer her very sternly, "Because they are hungry and their children are hungry." By these actions, Louise felt that her dad practiced Christianity even though he never attended church regularly. Louise told us that her favorite minister went overseas during World War II with a Jew, a Catholic, and a Protestant team to boost the morale of the soldiers. "That is Christianity to me," she avowed with conviction.

As we settled in the living room, Louise sat at her baby grand piano and spontaneously played long, sentimental songs for us like "Shine on Harvest Moon," "Four-Leaf Clover," and "My Dear." When one of us requested a song by title, Louise's facial expression recaptured the song's mood and feeling as she played it for us by ear. We asked her about "Deep Purple," for which the sheet music was prominently displayed on her piano. She proudly told us about a student whom she felt she had inspired when she taught piano. Louise recalled the moment she asked Carla, her student, to play "Deep Purple" while she stood by her side and listened intently. "I just let her play, and she played with tremendous feeling." Louise remembers that Carla looked up at her after finishing, and commented that she had made three or four mistakes. Louise told us that she vividly remembers her response to Carla as though it were yesterday. She said, "Carla, you have a gift from God. Don't let anyone change you. Those few sour notes don't matter and mistakes can be corrected. You felt every note that you played." Louise recalled that she had recently run into Carla's mother who gratefully told Louise of the impact she had had on her daughter. Louise told us, "I bet that was the day when Carla knew that I understood her." At ninety-two years of age, Louise still has the gift of bringing joy through her music, her long slender fingers gliding down the keyboard, her body swaying, and her left foot keeping time to the sounds of her heartfelt playing.

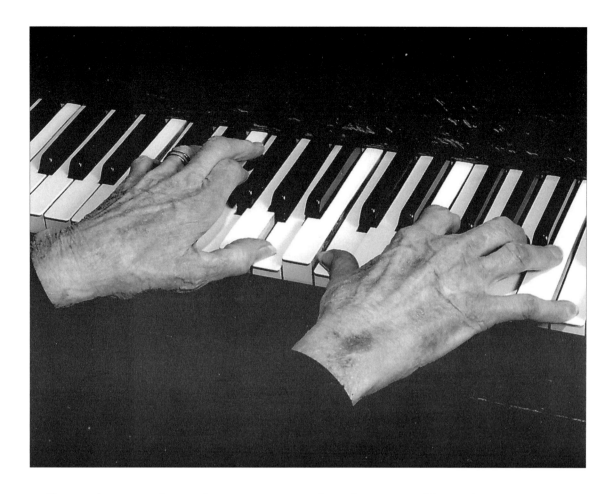

She was happy to share other memories involving her music. (Coinciden-
tally, her last name, Fogelsanger, translates into "bird singer" in German.)
Louise described an experience she had at Mayo Clinic in Minnesota when
she was eighty-seven years old. She sat down at a beautiful, stately grand piano
in the balcony of the hospital. As she began to play, people gathered around
her. She hoped that perhaps her gentle playing would provide a spiritual and
healing connection for all the patients and medical personnel listening. Louise stated that all of a sudden, one person from the crowd who recognized
her from the past called out, "Louise, let her rip like you can!" She was happy

to comply, and suddenly old jazz and ragtime songs came bellowing out of the stately grand piano. Louise recalls that faces in the crowd were ecstatic as folks moved rhythmically with the music. Even though her ragtime playing might not have been appropriate in that prestigious hospital, there was a part of her that knew deep down it might bring comfort to those around her. That memory remains precious to her to this day.

Louise's lifelong passion for music stems from her youth. Her siblings, one sister and one brother, were ten or more years younger, and she spent most of her days alone. The piano became her best friend. Her father soon recognized his daughter's extraordinary musical gifts. Louise played for various assemblies all through her high school days, with everyone enjoying her marvelous talent.

In the wintertime during the Depression years, folks from all around would bring their instruments to her father's country store. The group would gather around an old box stove to play country music. Louise loved these times, and it always inspired her to learn more instruments. She taught herself the harmonica, and she remembers hiding in the barn when only eight years old and practicing until she played it like second nature.

She told us about Drum Hall, where the high school kids congregated on weekends. Two boys from the high school formed a jazz band, and they desperately wanted Louise to play with them because of her incredible musicality. Her mother was very strict and stern, however, and would not let her play in that band. Louise admitted that she would go with her father to his country store, and he would let her "sneak away" to Drum Hall and practice with the band. Her mother never found out. On other occasions, Louise would ride with her father when he had meetings with bankers nearby, and he would drop her off at Drum Hall so she could play with the band. She states, "That's why I loved my dad. He had so many good qualities. He was tolerant and he had understanding for my love of music." His willingness to let her defy her mother's stern rules contributed to Louise's lifelong passion for the piano, and she has made every effort to have this "generosity of spirit" with her own piano students.

Louise has a lot of wonderful advice for young people: "Be considerate, look at things as a whole, practice tolerance." Almost every aspect of her life is informed by this approach, including her attitudes toward premarital sex, abortion, marijuana, and gay marriage. When asked to comment on these controversial issues, Louise replied simply, "I'm not running other people's business. I might be against something, but who am I to tell somebody what to do?"

Regarding friends, Louise shared that she has a few who are really close. "A true-blue friend is someone who can keep a secret and to whom you can pour out your troubles and it goes no further. I wish I had more male friends—I get starved for men's fellowship. It isn't sex," says ninety-two-year-old Louise, "I just speak men's language more than women's."

When we asked to what she attributes her longevity, she quickly replied, "I think people live longer if they have a good attitude and treat one another with respect. My mother lived to be ninety-six, and my father was eighty-nine when he passed. I really believe in chiropractic care and drive a little over an hour to my chiropractor's office. I am one of their oldest patients, and truly believe I wouldn't be here today without them. I also have a strong faith and believe in broad-minded charity. I came right out of the sticks in southeast Missouri, but I knew about truthfulness, consideration, and tolerance. I owe my father for living these truths, particularly evident during the Depression, and have tried to emulate his examples by living a long and meaningful life."

When asked about her impressions of kids today, Louise definitely had an opinion to share. "Children today don't know how to spend money.

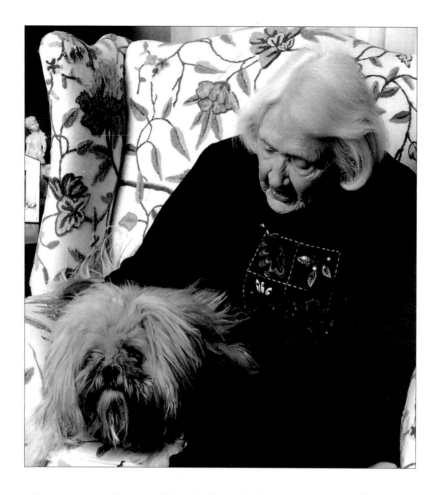

Parents just shower these kids, and they can't even afford it. I didn't shower my children with unnecessary things. When we owed money on our house, I showed the children that we were paying for it first. I put our expenses on a sheet of paper and showed them. Also, get children in 4-H clubs, music, and sports. Then they won't have time to sit in front of the TV."

Louise held strong views about current fashions: "I think it is horrible how young people dress today. First of all, parents pay a lot for clothes, and there is nothing to them. Kids go by labels and they compete with others. I don't approve of girls wearing short shorts to school. I think girls should wear a dress, skirt, or nice slacks and a blouse. If I had a daughter, they wouldn't show their skin, and I don't see any low-cut tops that are really pretty anyway. My feelings about boys—they have a waistline, put a belt around it."

We asked Louise if she had any regrets. After thinking for a time, she said, "The only regret I have is marrying for the second time and blending families. I love my stepson, but there were too many challenges at times. I also think it is best to avoid divorce if there are children. I've seen broken homes and it marks children in some way. They usually never come out of it like they do when the mother and father stay together."

As we continued to chat, she told us more about her accident and how wonderful it was that her son Larry came to stay with her while she recuperated. "You can't get a lot of sons to come from New York and stay with you for a couple of months. I told him that I'd get along, but he stays anyway." Louise's appreciation for these acts of loyalty, sacrifice, and kindness was also learned early from her father, his most meaningful legacy to her.

Leaving Louise's home in Casey, a central Illinois community of 3,500, we saw miles of rich farmland and an occasional farmhouse and grain storage bin in the distance. The simple beauty of this scenery seemed to provide the perfect finale for a glorious afternoon filled with the sounds and memories of Louise's music.

OSBORNE MUNROE

The Reverend Osborne George Munroe radiated a sense of calm. Perhaps it was because he grew up in the Bahama Islands where he was surrounded by green water and white sandy beaches that sparkled like diamond chips. Osborne, as he likes to be called, came to the United States in 1942, but he grew up on Ragged Island and in Nassau and still considers himself a Bahamian. He has kept this feeling of serenity from the days when he lived with the hills and trees of the island behind him and the ocean extending endlessly ahead.

Osborne's birth-mother and godmother were very close friends. "My godmother couldn't have children, so she asked my birth-mother a heartfelt question. If her next baby were a boy, would she give her the honor of raising him. My mother graciously agreed, and that is how it came to pass that my godparents raised me." He called his birth-mother Sister and his birth-father Mr. Munroe. Osborne played with his biological siblings and they knew the situation, accepted it, and remained close to him. Even though he was given more material things because his godparents were more well-to-do, his siblings were never jealous. "My birthparents and godparents were just so good at understanding things, and raised us with such an appreciation for one another," he said.

Osborne's godfather was a bandmaster on the island and taught him how to play many different instruments and to appreciate big band, jazz, and classical music. Osborne started playing the organ in church when he was eight years old. He would sit on his godmother's lap and play while she worked the pedals below. "My godparents were Seventh-Day Adventist, but they never stopped me from going to a Protestant church." Unfortunately, during this period of time, Osborne lost two fingers. He was playing with what he thought was a cap for a pencil. He started digging the insides out and hit gunpowder, which exploded. It was the same week his saxophone

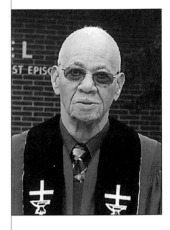

AGE: 88
"Have respect for everyone. Don't have hatred in your heart."

Authors' Reflection:
"It's the small things you do in life that count. Do something when someone least expects it."

37

and clarinet were delivered to him, so Osborne could never play those instruments. He did, however, persevere and ultimately learned how to play the French horn, trombone, trumpet, tuba, and organ.

As we continued talking, Osborne reminisced, "My daily life as a child consisted of going to school in one big building. Each grade was separated, but we were all together. After school my friends and I would play baseball, basketball, and then head to the ocean to surf or swim. The sun was almost always shining. I think it does make a difference in a person's mood being surrounded by this beauty in nature." He remembered several hurricanes and boarding up the house and riding out the storm. "There was always a calm before the storm," Osborne reflected.

Osborne told us that when he was growing up on the island, all of the families had their own gardens where they grew all the vegetables they ate. Along with fresh produce, grits, and fresh fish, they ate rice every day—it was a staple. Osborne related with a nostalgic smile that his godmother, who was a French woman, was a wonderful cook. He said that the special aroma of her cooking reached him all the way at school, and he could always identify it. "She could take something little and make it elaborate." Osborne's godfather made his living by fishing and selling sea salt. Like many of their neighbors, Osborne's godfather had a big pond that could be filled with seawater. He described a process by which the water evaporated and salt from the seawater would crystallize on top. His godfather would then "rake the salt in." Depending on how long the salt stayed on top of the water, it would be sold as a coarse, medium, or fine grade; a longer time on the water resulted in coarser-grained salt. Most of his godfather's salt was sold to Cuba, Haiti, and other surrounding islands, and the rest was used to cure the fish he caught. "We hung the fish out to dry just like we hang laundry in this country. My godfather would take that fish to Haiti and exchange it for food." He also remembered using kerosene lamps, as they had no electricity on the island.

Musical interests permeated Osborne's life. In addition to his early musical experiences with his godmother, he also played in a musical association as a young adult. He remembered two of these groups, one in the Bahamas and one in Miami, Florida. Each year the two groups competed with one another. One year when Osborne went to Miami with a friend, he decided to stay and volunteer for the United States Army. He was excused from combat during World War II because he played in the band. While stationed at an Air Force base in the Midwest, Osborne fell in love with a young woman. He shared a Bahamian saying that "one's first love is your main love." Everything was fine with the relationship until his girlfriend's aunt discovered their plans to marry. Their marriage never materialized. "I was truly in love with this woman, and I never had that feeling after that even though I dated several women. I remained single throughout my life and still have a picture of my first love," he confided. Osborne had planned to return to the islands after his tour of duty, but because both of his godparents had died while he was away, he decided to remain in the U.S.

We asked Osborne what prompted him to go into the ministry. He relayed to us that he had never attended church on the military base, but went to church in a city nearby. While attending that church, Osborne befriended an older woman who invited him to her home where he would read Bible scriptures. This friend strongly suggested that he should go into the ministry as she felt this was his true calling. While working for the Peoria Eastern Railroad and the University of Illinois, Osborne pursued the ministry and acquired many certificates pertaining to his ministerial education, earning the title of Reverend. He was also proud of the fact that during his work history he was the first black man hired at a Drivers License Bureau in his hometown.

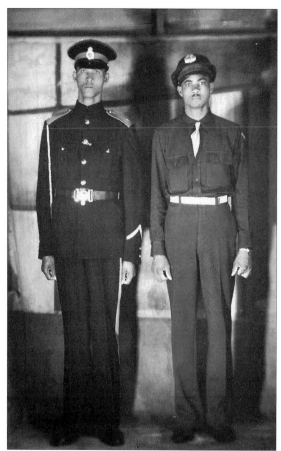

Osborne (right) with brother.

When visiting with Osborne, we always appreciated his hearty laugh and spontaneous humor. During one of the interviews, he turned on his favorite TV show, "The Steve Harvey" program, and we watched it together. Kim and I will never forget the scene in which the three of us sat and laughed until we ached. Sharing laughter created a strong feeling of friendship between us.

Presently, Osborne loves tending his roses and welcomes visitors to his garden, inviting them to be sure to pick a rose. He also enjoys bird-watching in his backyard. "I love to sit outside in the summer and watch them. Sometimes they will even get really close to me. They depend on me for food, and

I don't disappoint them," he said. "I also like to read Bible scriptures during the day and go to my church periodically to play the organ."

Sometimes Osborne mentors underprivileged kids. He still has a friendship with a man he mentored as a child, who calls him Dad. "I am proud to be alive and able to help others. I love children and older people. They seem to be honest, whereas the younger people tell you what you want to hear." Osborne remarked that he does get lonely and wishes there were more support groups for seniors with special interests such as music.

One of his regrets in life is that he didn't get more schooling. He had wanted to study to qualify for the Signal Corps in the military. Toward the end of our interview, he shared his advice to the younger generation: "Go to somebody's church. Have respect for everyone. Don't have hatred in your heart. Stay in school and get a good education. Most importantly, remember to pay attention to the small things. If you love somebody, it is always good to surprise him or her and not wait for a certain holiday. Meet them at the door with a rose. Small things are what grow up to be large and treasured."

LUCY GRAY

As we walked down the hall, we knew instantly which apartment was Lucy's by the handsome iron knocker and the antique pedestal standing by her door. We were aware that Lucy had been an antique dealer, and the interior and exterior of her apartment clearly reflected her love and appreciation of timeless treasures.

Lucy's apartment faces southwest, and as we sat down in her living room, the sun shining brightly through her big picture window highlighted the oriental rugs and beautiful antique furniture. She sat in her special chair near the picture window and the cabinet where she keeps all of her scrapbooks, old newspaper clippings, pictures, and anything that she deems really important.

Lucy candidly told us that she had definite ideas about various subjects, and was eager to share them with us. We decided to let her talk freely for hours on end, and her story unraveled as a stream of consciousness. Our questions became immaterial, and we proceeded to divide Lucy's "words of wisdom" into categories for our readers, gathering them into the special topics she wished to explore and a long reminiscence of events in her remarkable life.

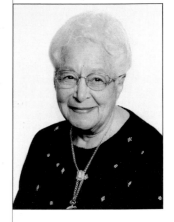

AGE: 93
"At night we would cut out paper dolls and tell stories around the kitchen table."

God and Life

With the wisdom and serenity of a great philosopher, Lucy reflected on her life. Although her attitude was generally optimistic, she initially began talking about people that have a poor quality of life. "I believe there are times when people would be better off not being here." With a puzzled look, she said that she doesn't understand why God lets some people live when they have such a poor quality of life. "Even at ninety-three," she said, "I feel when I get to the place where I can't take care of myself or help someone, I don't want to live anymore. But I'm not complaining, I am very thankful. Every day and every morning that I don't have any pain, I thank God." She

Authors' Reflection:
"Being poor has nothing to do with money. It has everything to do with the presence or absence of love."

43

emphasized this and glanced up as though she were looking at God and thanking Him.

Chuckling and with a big smile, she said, "I get up in the morning and grunt and groan for a minute. As far as suffering goes, my only problems are my hearing and my balance. The doctor told me that there is no cure for my hearing and no pill for my balance. I am thankful that I have lived this long, and I'm not afraid to die. I do tell my family that I'm not having a funeral. I don't want anyone to come and say, 'Doesn't she look nice? Doesn't she look natural?'" Lucy laughed very loudly at her comments at this point. "What else is there to say?"

Friendship

Friendship is very important to Lucy, and she feels that everyone should have at least one friend. "I have two friends I can depend on. When you get old, it is hard to find a friend. If you find an older friend, well we have deficiencies, so you can't be as friendly as when you were young." Lucy laughed a little as if she were speaking of herself. "I also think someone my age should have a young person for a friend. I have two young friends who are just absolutely dear to me. They call me almost every day. I feel older people should have a place where they feel safe, and I think places like where I live are so good. You used to have to move in with a friend or relative that didn't want you. They would take you in, but it wasn't always a comfortable situation. I thank God for places like my retirement village where people can go and be cared for and feel safe. That's the reason I'm here. At my age I felt I needed security, and I feel very secure here. Living with your family is OK if that's agreeable to all, but I think it puts a big burden on a young family to have to take care of their parents."

Pets and Older People

"In my opinion, animals are something to talk to and love." Lucy said that this was especially true in a place as quiet as her apartment. "I could go downstairs and talk to a lot of elderly people, but I think one feels closer to an animal at this stage of life. I once had a kitty cat for four years to keep me company." Lucy said that she loved her cat but that eventually she had to find another home for her. "My kitty would jump in front of me when I would get up at night. So many people fall at my age and get broken bones. Unfortunately, people don't heal well at this age. I take calcium and drink lots of milk, but for safety reasons I gave her to an elderly bachelor. I gave him all the equipment." She laughed heartily, thinking of the litter box, scoop, and favorite toys. Lucy continued, "I miss her terribly. I love dogs as well, but you have to walk a dog every day if you are a diligent and caring owner. I've had collies and they would look at me like they knew exactly what I was saying. They were good company and I think all older people should have a pet of some kind."

Growing Up

"We were a family of six children—three girls and three boys. My father was a laborer and we were very poor, but we were a happy family. We didn't know we were poor until we saw the other kids doing different things, but we were always busy in different ways. I will never forget the time somebody gave us a Victrola. We had hardwood floors and we danced to that Victrola. I can still remember how much fun we had dancing. I can't imagine any children not having a Victrola and not being able to dance like we did. One day we got a player piano, and I honestly don't remember how we got that, as we were so poor.

"We were able to go to movies once in a while. There was a streetcar, but it only ran on one street in the town. We never had the money to ride the streetcar, so we walked everywhere. Another fun remembrance was when our town finally got streetlights, which were located in the middle of the streets. The children in the neighborhood would meet at night under the light in the corner and tell ghost stories. I don't think children today know what real ghost stories are." Lucy reflected in her body language just how scared the kids would really get. "Sometimes the kids would tell stories so scary that we were almost afraid to go home," she said with a grin.

"Another vivid childhood memory was going to fish at the lake with our mother. My mother loved to fish. Mother would fix us a sandwich and some water, and we would all walk to the lake, which was about three or four miles away. It was our fun. We couldn't wait to walk to the lake and watch our mother fish. Activities at night included cutting out paper dolls and telling stories around the table. Thinking back and knowing now how poor we were monetarily, I wonder how we survived.

"Everybody in town had a garden with lots of fruit trees. We had a pear tree, two apple trees, a cherry tree, a peach tree, and a big grape arbor. My grandmother was an excellent cook and made really good pies. She also made the best sauerkraut you've ever tasted. We canned all summer because we didn't have freezers back then. We canned everything—lots and lots of fruit. My grandmother had a cellar where she would put her sweet and Irish potatoes for the winter. We also ate a lot of beans and cornbread. In the wintertime, we ate a lot of rabbit, LOTS of rabbit. My dad was never a hunter, but our neighbors were and shared everything with us.

"I can remember my grandmother trying to show me how to kill a chicken. Cousin Lucy would have a kettle of boiling water that she had gotten from the well. Grandmother would say, 'You should never make a chicken suffer.' She knew right where to put her thumb." Lucy took her hand and held it up in the position that she had seen her grandmother do so many times, contorting her fingers as if she were grabbing a chicken. She twisted her hand just one time. "She knew just how to pull the neck off without causing the chicken to suffer. A lot of people would do this another way." Lucy continued, twirling her hand as if she were wringing the neck of a chicken, "But my grandmother never did that. Even though I was taught the proper way, I could never kill a chicken. I remember how she put them down in the well to cool.

"My father laid the first brick roads. The workers laid bricks by hand, but that was a good job for the summer. The company provided us a tent with a wooden floor and dad had a truck. My grandmother cooked for the laborers and that is why our family was able to travel with my dad. We would pitch the tent any place he was working, and that's the way we lived one summer. We were healthy and happy." (Lucy emphasized *happy*.) "We would make a fire with sticks and cook over the fire with one big kettle. We ate lots of soup and soup beans. Dad traveled all around Illinois, but mainly he laid the brick roads in southern Illinois. The bricks were only laid on one side of the road years ago; some of the roads are still around. Also, I remember my father laying brick highways.

"During my childhood, I vividly remember the only time that I got a new dress. There was a lady that lived on the corner who was a seamstress that made each of the girls in our family a new dress at Easter time. I wish I still had that dress that left such an impression on me. It was the most beautiful dress I had ever seen—a pale blue dress with a cape collar. I think they called them Bertha collars. It was a simple dress, but when she put that collar on the dress, it was the first time I really felt dressed up. I can see that dress right now…." Lucy gazed off in the distance, remembering and picturing the dress in her mind.

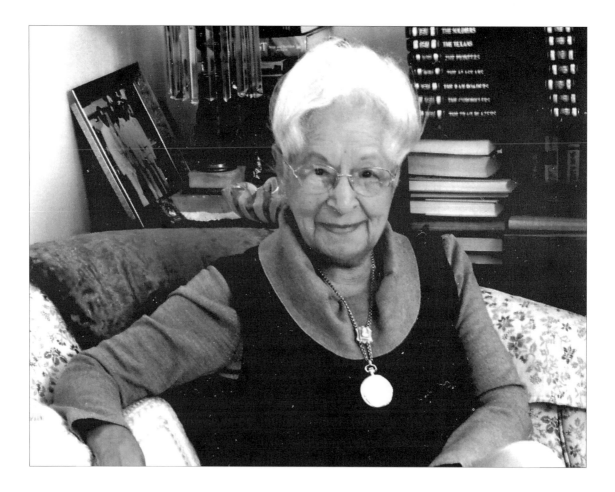

"We thought our Christmas was good because Santa Claus always brought us one gift. He always brought lots of candy, apples, and oranges, and we each got one special gift. So yes, Christmas was a happy time, a very happy time. My grandmother cooked for us at Christmas. She made wonderful cornbread. I can't think of anything special—everything she cooked was so good. My grandmother lived to be in her seventies. I write down a lot of things I remember and put them in a book. I don't know if any of my children or grandchildren will appreciate this book, but they are going to get it anyway! My mother died when she was in her sixties—people got older faster when I was growing up, probably because of the hard physical work that was required and no advanced medical technology."

Lucy reminisced about "Cousin Lucy Jenkins," who was a cousin or a "person we might have just called a cousin…. She was part Indian and I was named after her." Lucy's voice became very quiet as she described her cousin. "Lucy Jenkins was very artistic and made beautiful quilts. I don't know what happened to them after she passed away. She was a very quiet person, and I always liked to talk to her. I knew that she loved me." Although Cousin Lucy was a loner and considered different from others, Lucy was drawn to her, to her artistic qualities and her thoughtfulness. There was a quiet presence about her that she appreciated. Even her eccentricities seemed to be something special. Unfortunately, Lucy reported that she didn't have any pictures of her cousin. She commented that she wasn't sure if this woman ever had a picture taken.

"My father's mother also made beautiful quilts. In those days women sat down together and that was their entertainment. Nothing was thrown away. Every scrap of any material that was not worn out would be saved and made into patchwork quilts. Everyone had lots of quilts because that's what we used to cover up with to keep warm. They were all lined with a cotton blanket. We had a coal stove in the corner of the dining room where we lived. All of us would sit around the dining-room table at night with just one light." Lucy looked up as she described their one light—an electric cord coming down from the ceiling with a bulb at the end. "In the wintertime, my father would say, and I will never forget, 'This is the last lump of coal for the night; when this is gone, you'd better go to bed.' So we would all huddle around the stove to get warm and then jump in bed. We had to ration not only our coal but also everything we had.

"Even though the rooms in our home were large, our home only consisted of a kitchen, one bedroom, a dining room, and a living room. Boys and girls slept together. If you got sleepy, you just crawled into bed. If you had company it was the same way. If there wasn't enough room in the bed,

you slept on the floor." Lucy chuckled, "I don't think children sleep on the floor anymore, do they?" She continued, "We knew boys were boys and girls were girls, but we only had two beds. My brother and I slept on the couch in the dining room for years until we were big kids. We never thought anything about it. Now every time you pick up a magazine or watch television you realize there is no more innocence anymore. We finally learned that there was a difference, but we were twelve or thirteen years old before we stopped sleeping with our brother and sisters. Now boys and girls don't even have the same room—they are not innocent anymore. I don't know whether that is good or bad.

"I wish they would do something to eliminate so much TV in households. It is not a good influence on our children or our adults. Children now have TVs in their rooms where they sleep, and you can't control what they are watching. Certainly, the children aren't to blame, but I do think that they have lost their innocence much too early.

"The beds we did own were made of feather ticks [mattresses]. Sometimes we had straw ticks. My kids laugh, but we had straw ticks although they didn't last as long as the feather ticks. Feather ticks will last forever. Cousin Lucy gave me two feather ticks when I married, and my husband and I slept on them for years. In fact, when I had that couch recovered [she pointed to her couch with the wooden claw feet and curved back], I had the upholsterer put those feather ticks in it. Those feathers in my couch are from the ducks and geese that my cousin Lucy raised so they are probably over 100 years old.

"Our house didn't have an indoor toilet. We had a three-seater toilet outhouse. There were two for the adults and one for the little ones." She put her hand lower to the floor to show the different heights of the seats. Lucy asked us if we had ever seen an outhouse. "We called them toilets, but today they call them outhouses. We used magazines and newspapers for toilet paper." Lucy laughed with a hint of embarrassment when she told us about the magazines and newspapers. "Sears and Roebuck catalogs were a great gift!" Lucy recalled.

Lucy said that, for the most part, she and her family enjoyed good health. "Sometimes poor people are healthier than wealthier people. We all had the childhood diseases such as measles and chicken pox, but we weren't really sick, we were just quarantined. The only time I can remember having a doctor is when my mother would have a baby. When I got older and was in high school, I had a sore throat and was terribly sick. I stopped in the doctor's office and told him I didn't have any money, but I was very sick. Everybody knew everyone in a small town like ours, so he gave me some medicine. That is the only time I remember going to the doctor."

Lucy talked about the kind of discipline she experienced as a child. "My mother would ask us to get a switch—our own switch. If you got one that was too little, she would say, 'Now you know that's not what I want.' She left subtle marks on us. If you leave a mark on your child today, your child can have you arrested. That's brutal," she said with anger in her voice. "There were a lot of marks on us and it didn't hurt us a bit." Lucy lay back in her chair and really started laughing. "We were all spanked—not with a paddle, but with a switch. If we did something that was really wrong, we would have to get a switch from the pear tree. I look back and I think it was probably due to its being a stronger tree. When my mother would demand that we get a switch off the pear tree, I knew we were in for some real punishment."

When we asked Lucy if she remembers experiencing racism when she was growing up, she said, "No, but as I think back I suppose there was. Now that they make a big issue out of racism, it is a big issue. It was called segregation not racism in my time. Just the churches were segregated, but that was a choice. We had two beautiful Negro churches—a Methodist and a Baptist

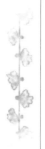

Church—but they don't exist anymore. We felt that is wasn't segregation, just separate religious teachings. We all go to the same place; we just have different ways of teaching and learning. It was a wonderful time because everybody went to church. Church was a spiritual place where you met your friends on Sunday. We had church twice a day on Sunday," Lucy said with strong feeling. "That was our fellowship—everybody knew everybody, and we had a sense of community. We all knew everyone's family—rich or poor, black or white."

Nevertheless, Lucy recalled a time in the 1940s when "Negro soldiers on scholarships came to Urbana [IL] to attend college. Five Negro men came here, but weren't allowed to stay on the campus and they couldn't even eat at a popular local diner. If they wanted anything, they had to send a white man in to get it. A few Negro women and I got together and decided to take these students into our homes. I lived in Urbana at the time and kept three boys. We fixed a room upstairs where the boys slept. We charged them $3.00 a month for their room and board. We kept them all through college; their mothers would send food to them on weekends. That was a wonderful experience—we were just a family. They all graduated with honors. I used to hear from the boys often, and they would bring their wives and children to visit me. Two or three weeks ago, I heard from one of them who is still living. He is eighty-eight years old now."

Marriage, Home, and Family

"Being a friend is the most important ingredient in a successful marriage. My husband was the best friend I ever had in my life." Lucy started choking up as she mentioned her husband and her lips were quivering. As Lucy reflected on her close relationship with her husband, her head hung low. "He was truly a friend. Anytime I had a question or a problem, I could go to my husband. I was not afraid to tell him anything. Even if I saw a handsome man, I would make some kind of comment and he would laugh." She continued to smile as she talked about her husband. Lucy felt that a lot of women couldn't say those kinds of things to their husbands. "He was my hero. He loved me dearly, and I could go to him with anything I said, did, or thought. I was eighteen and he was twenty-six when we married."

Lucy reminisced about how she and her husband met. "There used to be dances every Saturday night in the park. They were held in a tent with a wooden platform for the floor. There were five girls and only one Negro boy in our high school. Most of the time the girls danced together. One Saturday, some boys discovered that there were some girls in our town, so we finally had some boys with whom to dance. I met my husband at one of these dances. I knew my husband about six months before I married him. Sadly, he died in his forties."

Lucy told about the house she owned for twenty-five years. She said, "I was driving by one day and realized it was being auctioned off. I was on my way to work so I stopped. I had admired the house for many years. It was very run down, and the auctioneer wondered why anyone would want the house, especially a woman." Lucy won the bid, and many friends pitched in to help her fix it up. It was in bad shape and infested with rats. Friends washed walls, scrubbed floors, and painted, and no one expected any compensation for this work. Lucy furnished the house with her favorite antiques from the store she owned. When she finished decorating, hundreds of people from all over the city came to see her home. There were pictures in the paper, and it felt, she said, like a big debutante ball. She was proud that the house was so beautiful. In her wonderful dining room hung the original crystal chandelier. Then Lucy started on the yard. Again people came to help because they were so happy someone was refurbishing the old house and cleaning up the yard. She hosted fundraisers in her home for her church and its missionaries.

If someone wanted to have a social event or gathering, they were welcome to use Lucy's home and enjoy magnificent garden parties in the spring and summer. For twenty-five years Lucy lived in this home filled with "character." Then, when she couldn't take care of the yard or the house any longer, she moved to the apartment where we met her. She has been in her present location for six years. Sadly, the people who bought the house cut down all the trees, shrubs, and flowers. Lucy was quite pensive as she described how sad it was to see her beloved home with no flowers and no lush vegetation.

Lucy has one son, two grandchildren, and eleven great-grandchildren. She says her great-granddaughter calls her every week. Her son lives nearby, but Lucy and he are estranged. She said she just prays over the whole situation now. She prays for him and for herself every day. "He needs prayer and so do I. We all live different lives, and that is just the way we are—we can't all be the same."

Life Today

Lucy commented that she has gained sixteen pounds since she moved into her apartment and had never weighed more than 110 pounds in her whole life. "I'm saving all of my clothes because I hope to get back to my desired weight. I don't go shopping very often—only if I have to," Lucy laughed. "I'm not as active as I used to be, so I quit eating three meals a day; I just have one meal a day, except for breakfast when I have one piece of toast so I can take my pills. All old people have to take pills. I asked the doctor, 'Why do I have to take all these pills?'" Her voice rose in a humorous tone while describing the question to her doctor. Laughing heartily, she continued, "He said, 'to stay alive and stay healthy.' So I take them. Everybody takes medicine today. I never took any medicine for the majority of my life. There were only two items in our medicine cabinet—aspirin and castor oil. My mother and father always knew if we were constipated, so we were given castor oil. It was something that you automatically were given at Christmastime because we ate lots of candy and cookies. So we all had to have a dose of castor oil to 'clean us out.' Old people used to think that our systems needed to be cleaned out, and those are the words they used to describe it.

"There are a lot of older people who don't have the money to live in a place like mine." Lucy said that she was thankful that she was healthy enough to work hard and save for retirement. She was very thankful that she had lots of friends, loved working, and enjoyed people. "That's what made it possible for me to have the care that I am enjoying today. Education helps you make more money—that was impossible at my age where I grew up. I'm not truly happy here, although I thank God every day for a place like this where I feel secure. This isn't the way I intended to end my life. However, I didn't know I was going to live this long either. I thought I would have my husband. You don't always have a choice."

Lucy tries to maintain a positive attitude every morning when she awakens. "I exercise every morning before I get out of bed! I exercise my arms [Lucy started moving her arms around in a circle] and legs, and then I get down on the floor and exercise again. If I didn't I would really be stiff. When the weather is nice I walk about four blocks. There is a sidewalk all around this building, but I walk on the street—that way I know if I have gone four blocks. I exercise every day either on the floor or in bed."

Lucy's Words of Wisdom

When asked to comment about war, Lucy responded with conviction that it is simply ridiculous. "As smart as we are supposed to be, we shouldn't have to kill one another to settle disputes. Our population is more educated now than it has ever been, supposedly, but evidently the education is not helping

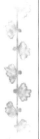

because we are killing each other. I will probably not live to see the end of our present war, but I suffer in silence thinking about the families that are affected as their loved ones serve overseas."

Lucy feels that not only are we killing innocent people in our present situation at war, but we are also "killing" our environment. "Guns aren't the only weapons in war. Our present generation of people is not concerned enough about our environment, and our air and food are being poisoned."

She believes strongly that one should live each day to the fullest, because tomorrow is not promised. Lucy seldom watches TV, but she does watch the news. She loves to look out her picture window, but worries about all of the new construction. "People are living better than we ever did in our day, but they don't pay attention to values, environment, and friendships. At ninety-three years of age, I remember how things used to be and how comfortable we were. We were happy without realizing how poor we were. Now people only seem to be happy if they have lots of possessions. When I grew up it wasn't what you had, but what friends you had. One felt blessed if you had family and friends."

Lucy abhors the way young people dress today and holds strong opinions. She said she thinks it is a disgrace and that something should be done about it. With a steadily rising voice, she said, "I was somewhere the other day and the girls all had on these little tight pants and their belly buttons were showing. Now, in my opinion, that is not good. It is a different world, but I think that young people are exposing too much. That is one reason these young girls are having babies when they are still babies themselves. Sex seems to be the way of life, so young girls are exposing themselves and the boys are taking advantage of it. You can't blame them—it is our culture. I don't care how much work the church does or how hard your mother tries to teach you right from wrong, the youngsters look at TV and magazines and this is what they see. There is no innocence anymore. I feel sorry for this generation, and I feel sorry for the children who are having babies when they are so young." Lucy maintains that the media exploits young people; she hopes that the pendulum swings back in the twenty-first century and solid values are reinstated in our society.

Lucy sometimes asks her grandchildren why they want so much—why they have to have this and that. "I tell them we were raised with maybe a penny or two for Sunday school. If there was an ice-cream social or something maybe we would have a nickel. We never had any money—we didn't need it."

Lucy firmly advises young people to get a good education—all the education they can acquire. "I think it is so very, very important today. Life has changed so much, and the young are exposed to so many things that aren't wholesome and bring our society down. One needs a good education to live a better life."

We told Lucy how much we enjoyed her memories of her past and remarked that some of her stories seemed to overlap with those of other people we had interviewed. "Well," she declared, "these stories should be remembered."

As we concluded our conversation in her living room full of antiques and memories, Lucy remarked, "It is so much more fun talking about the good old days than talking about what is happening now. We had FUN."

CLIFF MYERS

At the age of 102, Clifford Myers burns his night-light until the wee hours of every morning as he lies in bed or on the couch reading his favorite novels by Zane Grey or Louis L'Amour. "Cliff" loves stories about the Old West. He knows the two authors lived in the West and understood firsthand what life in that part of the country was truly like. In addition to late-night reading, Cliff finds many things in life that are still fulfilling and satisfying. Other favorite pastimes are riding around town with his son, eating out, and watching TV shows such as "Andy Griffith," "Oprah," and the "Price is Right." He also finds time to talk to a special "lady friend" each night. He told us that he is scared to ask her to marry him, for fear she will say yes! This deadpan humor reflects Cliff's continued joy in living, even at the age of 102. Laughingly, he says that "one can lose his hair, one can lose his teeth, but one can never lose his sense of humor!"

Reminiscing about friends from his military days, Cliff remembers an older gentleman who once told him that he hoped to live a long time and "die laughing." Cliff obviously agrees with this philosophy, and maintaining a sense of humor has always been his trademark. During World War II, Cliff worked at the Crab Orchard ammunitions plant in Carbondale, Illinois. The plant manufactured 500-pound bombs. He recalls that his plant foreman walked up to him one day and said, "Cliff, do you see that whistle over there? If you ever see the plant catch on fire, go blow that whistle immediately." With a big grin, Cliff told us that he responded, "Sir, if there is ever a fire in this building, the only way that whistle will blow will be from the wind of my rear as I go by!"

Cliff has lived through five different wars. He has outlived three wives and has raised seven children. Unfortunately, one of his children died. Cliff states, "After the death of our child, I had to continue going on with life. A person doesn't have any problems, I realized, if you have your health and your children are healthy." Cliff told us he gave up smoking forty years

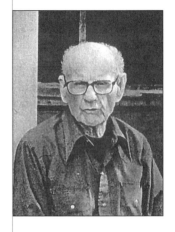

AGE: 102
"One can lose his hair, one can lose his teeth, but one can never lose his sense of humor."

Authors' Reflection:
"Your character is your most important attribute. It will follow you for life."

ago. He "talked" to his cigarettes for a week, and one day he laid his Lucky Strikes on the dashboard of his truck. Looking at the cigarettes, Cliff said, "I don't need you silly things anymore." From that point forward, he never smoked again.

Cliff loves recalling the "good old days." He remembers attending square dances, swimming in creeks, watching silent movies, playing board games such as Parcheesi and Chinese checkers, and playing outdoor games like Hide-and-Seek and Kick-the-Can. Cliff states, "Those were fun times and I will never forget them." Some of his most priceless memories relate to times when he rode his special horse, Dudley. He proudly relates that Dudley was the fastest horse in town. He and his friends would often take their horses to an open field to race, and although his friends' horses came close occasionally, no one ever beat Dudley.

Cliff's other most treasured memories revolve around selling produce, which he has done throughout his lifetime. Selling apples and peaches has been his vocation and avocation to the present day. This passion began when his father owned a nursery near a national forest. He recalls that he and his father took a ferry across the Mississippi River to get to markets where his father would sell apple trees. When Cliff began selling fruit, he traveled all over surrounding states to sell his produce. He is proud of the fact that he made four to five dollars a day during the Depression, when other men had jobs that paid barely a dollar a day. According to Cliff, all business transactions were done on a handshake, at a time in history when mutual trust was the standard. This tradition of selling fruit has continued with Cliff's son Frank helping him at his fruit stand each spring and summer. At one time Cliff drove all over southern Illinois and southeast Missouri selling fruit to feed his large family. Cliff has always lived by the rule, "Worry will kill you; hard work will pay the bills." His business now is limited to one local roadside stand, which is open every Friday morning during the spring and summer. He likes to brag about the fruit and the orchards from which the fruit is picked, and he always tells his customers that he "wouldn't sell anything he wouldn't want to buy himself." Because of his honesty and loyalty, Cliff now has third-generation customers. According to Frank, his father always offered money back or more produce if a customer was ever dissatisfied.

In his late eighties, Cliff took an interest in poetry, and he still loves to write, read, and recite poems. Frank does most of the selling at the produce stand these days, while Cliff visits with his regular customers and recites poetry to them. The first poem that we heard him recite was Longfellow's "The Children's Hour." We were sitting in his daughter's living room with his children and grandchildren, and the skill with which he recited the poem verbatim was very impressive. Cliff was happy to share some of his own poetry with us as well. One poem was written when he was watching people of different ethnicities, ages, and genders walk hurriedly through a busy airport at Phoenix. Cliff states, "I sat in the airport and thought about how dependent we really are on one another, and I wondered if people ever give much thought to this." The following poem is the result of Cliff's pondering that day:

While Waiting for My Flight

While waiting for my flight at the airport one day,
I started watching people winding their merry way.
Some were short and some were tall
And some were in between,
But one that looked just like me was nowhere to be seen.

I could not help but wonder what was their destination and
When they safely arrived there, what was their occupation?
They were probably doctors, lawyers and pretty nurses, too.

But, don't forget the farmer, who works from sun to sun
And no matter how hard he works, his work is never done.

Cliff's poem "Advice to Married Men," written on October 24, 2001 when Cliff was ninety-five years of age, is his favorite:

Advice to Married Men

My fellow friends and husbands,
I have some advice for you.
Now, I don't have all the answers,
But I do have quite a few.

And as we travel this Highway
Of Married Life together,
You'll encounter sunny skies,
And also, cloudy weather.

And always have the last word
As arguments appear.
But, Brother let it end this way
With a contrite "yes Dear."

And take her in your arms,
Look into her pretty eyes.
And though it may startle her,
And take her by surprise,

Just tell her sincerely
I love you sweetheart dear,
And may our love grow stronger
With every passing year.

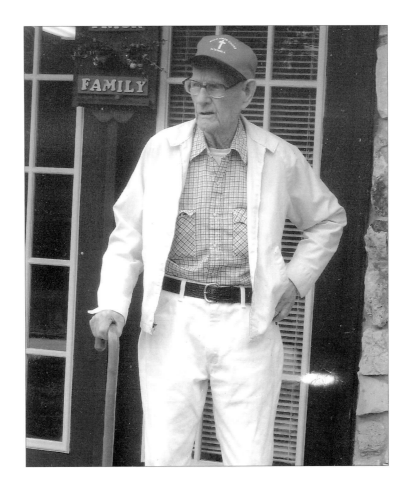

After reading this poem to us, Cliff looked up and said, "When you are truly happy in marriage, you are totally compatible and true to each other. You know you are in love when you don't want to be with anyone else."

At 102 years, Cliff Myers looks forward to the coming spring, when he hopes to accompany Frank to the same roadside stand. His son remarks, "He's out there because he can still do it, enjoy it, and show everyone that he can." There at the stand, Cliff hopes to shake hands once again with his loyal customers, tell some jokes, and recite his poetry—and, just perhaps, he'll sell a few peaches, too.

DAVIE HILL

Ninety-three-year-old Davie Hill is the matriarch of her family, a loving mother of three children, five grandchildren, and five great-grandchildren. "She is a woman whose wisdom exemplifies what life should be," Diane, her daughter, caretaker, and best friend, said proudly.

A typical day for Davie begins with coming to the Circle of Friends Center, where she reads and enjoys her talks with Robin, her favorite caretaker. She enjoys chatting throughout the day with her about their respective children and grandchildren. She gets great comfort from their conversations about past and present memories, although some are painful to recall, such as the death of Davie's husband at the young age of fifty-five. Davie likes listening to public broadcast radio and watching PBS documentaries. She loves books and especially relishes reading about African-Americans, such as Rosa Parks and Maya Angelou. Communication of all sorts, whether through books, conversations with others, or public broadcasting, keeps her living a happy, self-fulfilled life.

Davie enjoys talking about her past teaching career in the Head Start Program, and she explained to us how she became a teacher. She was caring for the children of a professor and his wife when they urged her to apply for a Head Start position. Although she had never taught in a formal setting and was reluctant to apply, she was hired. She states that teaching at Head Start changed her life. She feels blessed to have been in a position to share her wisdom and knowledge with children. "Every child has something to give, and I learned something from each child. Teaching children was the best part of my life." The highest compliment that Davie received was from a gentleman who resisted her impending retirement. He said, "Davie, you can't retire from teaching at Head Start because YOU ARE the Head Start program." Indeed, she gave her heart and soul to teaching for fifteen years.

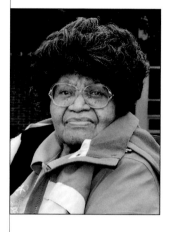

AGE: 93
"My advice to people in this generation is to have a strong relationship with the Lord."

Authors' Reflection:
"Spend lots of time with your children and engage them in various activities, large and small. Children learn from your example."

When we questioned Davie about the most important things she has passed on to her students, she immediately talked about the gardens they had planted together and the children's curiosity and excitement as things began to grow. The population of children in the school was quite diverse, and she loved that they came from all over the world. Davie recalls some "Indian children" wanting to know how vegetables end up in cans in the grocery store, so she planted vegetables, nurtured them until they ripened, and then prepared them for canning so that all the children could understand the process. She states, "I always took everything in my teaching a step further and related it to their immediate life." The children always helped Davie in the garden and expressed amazement and joy as they saw the fruits of their labor.

Davie's parents initiated the legacy of teaching by example. When she and each of her siblings reached the age of six, their mother showed them how to cook and sew. Davie's voice got animated as she described how her parents stood beside their children and taught them how to develop their own skills. She recalls memorable times when her mother and the children would walk through fields with high grass. They would pick berries to prepare homemade pies and cakes. Davie describes her mother actually beating the cake batter with her bare hands, as they didn't have mixers in those days. She and her siblings also loved learning how to crochet. They even learned to crochet brassieres, and she still has one that she made herself.

Her dad always talked and laughed with his children. He stood side by side with them as they learned to garden. He stressed turning over the soil before planting flowers or vegetables. She recalls, "Dad taught me how to plant and what to plant." She still cherishes pink roses—a tribute to her father who, she said, "had the biggest pink blooms." Her dad taught her to "always say a prayer before you plant a tree," and his words still echo in her memory.

Davie has many other clear memories of her childhood, most happy, a few humiliating. The girls played with dolls made of cornhusks and sewed doll clothes for them. Quilting was also a favorite pastime, and the ladies even made their own patterns. After the quilting was completed, the women stuffed the pieces with cotton. Davie's father would not let her mother pick any cotton, however, nor would he let her mother work for any "white folk." He maintained two jobs so that her mother could remain at home with her own family. She recalls her father saying, "I don't care how many white folk need help. If the white women need their floors scrubbed, let them get on their knees and scrub them." Growing up in the deep South, Davie witnessed many racial inequities. Because her father worked for the railroad, the family could ride free, but with one stipulation: they had to sit in the "Jim Crow" car, which rode behind the smoke. The movie *Jane Pitman* stands out in Davie's mind as a classic film. She has watched it repeatedly because at the end Jane had enough courage to walk up to the "white" people's water fountain, where she drank some water and declared: "That water tasted so good." The movie ends with those words. In spite of the inherent racial problems in the South that Davie experienced while growing up, she persevered, remained dignified, and harbors no bitterness or resentments.

Davie is very clear in offering advice on how to live a good life and expressing her views on contemporary issues such as sex before marriage, abortion, and dress codes of young women. "Sex before marriage is a taboo for me. I don't think couples should live together before marriage. There are some things that should be found out after marriage. Parents need to actively talk to their children about these kinds of issues as the children are growing up. If an unplanned pregnancy does occur and a woman is unable to care for her child, I would hope that she would consider making

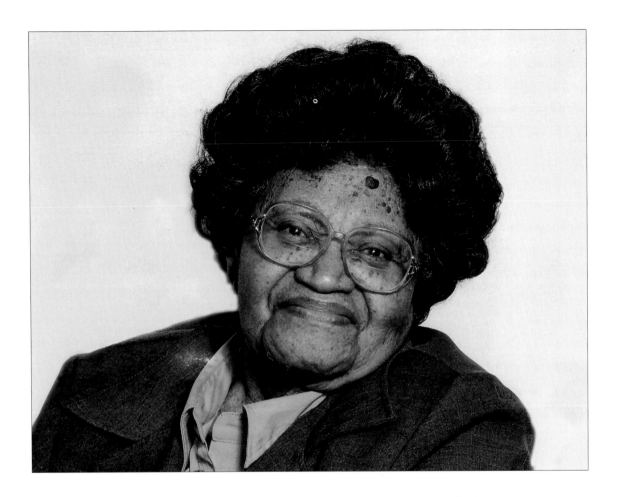

a plan of adoption." She also thinks that young girls dress too provocatively. "Again, I think parents should take the time and sit down with their daughters to discuss the consequences of dressing inappropriately. I also don't approve of young men wearing earrings and pants that fall to their knees. Talking to children at every stage of their development is key…. It appears to me that everyone in today's world is trying to be a big shot and be the one making the most money. My parents didn't dwell on making money, although they set a good example by having a strong work ethic. They taught us to have a strong faith in God. My advice to people in this generation is to have a strong relationship with the Lord. I credit the good Lord for watching over my family and me." Davie still sees friends at church, two of whom have been attending the same church as she has for sixty-eight years.

During our last interview, Davie shared a charm bracelet with us that was given to her by her grandson. The symbols of each charm represent the culmination of her teachings, and she realized that this gift summarized what she had always hoped would be her legacy to her family. These are her grandson's explanations presented to Davie along with the bracelet:

Grannie's Bracelet Links

Coffee Cup

I will always remember the smell of the coffee in the morning.
When I smelled coffee brewing, I knew it was time to get ready for school.
Even today when I smell coffee I think of you.

Thimble

This thimble reminds me of the many buttons
you sewed on our shirts because
Mama had to drive so far to get to work.
I thank you. We always looked fresh and neat.

Feet

You weren't there for my first steps, because you and Daddy Joe
Were in Liberia West Africa, but you and Mama took me,
Eddie and Taffie (our collie) on walks in the evening to
Look at the sun going down. We would get up early enough to see
the sun rise. We watched for rainbows after the rain. We still do.

Musical Note

*At night when I would get sleepy, I would sit in your lap and you would
Hum a tune as you rocked me to sleep only it would sound like a kazoo
against my ear. I loved the sound of it.*

Heart

*You have such a loving heart. I watch you talk to some of your parents
In Head Start. The parent came in very upset, but when you finished
talking to her about what she thought was a problem, she was
smiling, hugging and thanking you. I want to be the same way with
my basketball parents.*

Heaven

*If anyone is going to heaven Grannie, it will be you.
We are going to try to live our lives so we can be there
With you when our time comes.*

LLOYDE DEES

Lloyde Dees, whose early religious education was steeped in a fear-based dogmatic tradition, has now come full circle in his thinking. Believing in a beneficent and merciful God, Lloyde spends his daily life ministering to the needs of others in a nonjudgmental way.

At the age of eighty-eight, Lloyde serves as a parish visitor who calls on shut-ins, patients in the hospital, and people who are grieving because of the loss of a loved one. He also visits his homebound sister every day. He wants to know that at the end of his life he helped her as much as possible. One woman whom Lloyde visits told him how much she admires his goatee. He responded that he grew the beard because pulling on it makes him think better.

When Lloyde visits people in hospitals and nursing homes, he employs what he has found to be the most effective, greatest technique possible—to be an excellent listener. He doesn't preach, doesn't "sell" anything, and doesn't try to get them to tell him what is going on in their lives. Lloyde finds that, in general, when people do ask for his advice in solving a problem, they really are not seeking it. They just want someone to listen. People, in Lloyd's opinion, want to share information without being judged. This, he feels, is the real essence of religion, not adhering blindly to a certain dogma that everyone must believe. Lloyde tries to practice saying hello to everybody he sees, "searching for someone that maybe I need or who needs me." He feels strongly that human beings need one another. In his twenty-three years of serving as a visitor in people's homes and as a witness of God, many have told Lloyde what they believe, and then confided that they hope it is true. He feels that these people are trying to create a human God. He recognizes that our mind cannot grasp the infinite and recognize the reality of an all-powerful being. We really can't begin to comprehend the magnitude of such an understanding. "My personal prayer is that I will always be a good witness

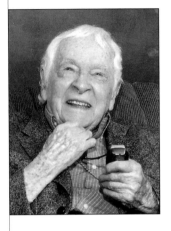

AGE: 88
"My buddies could never convince me at all that war was necessary. It doesn't solve anything except that it sets it up for the next war."

Authors' Reflection:
"Spiritual maturity is giving to others and letting go of your own wants and needs."

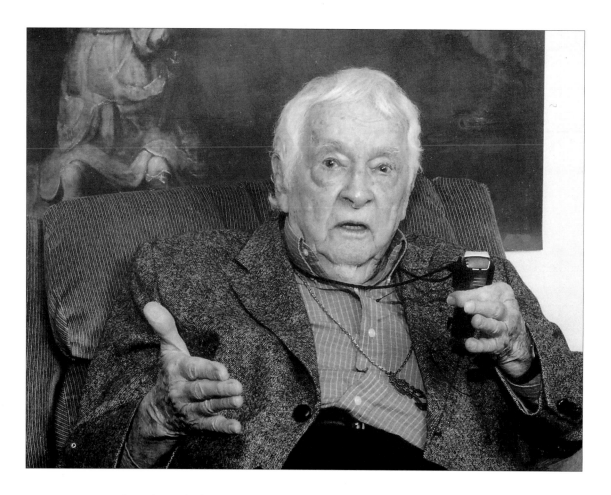

for what I believe. Nothing else really matters. I understand that people in our present society struggle because they feel someone is always looking over their shoulder expecting the terrorists to attack. So mistrust in the community is rampant. I don't worry about things like that. One can also find people who love you. And, one can never get enough of that. We all need each other."

One offshoot of his "visitation" practice is teaching an adult Sunday school class. Lloyde talked about the lesson he was preparing on the subject of controversy. "When I am teaching, I always hope to get feedback. You never really know how effective you really are. It haunts you." He holds that controversy should be welcome, as long as both parties are sincere and each respects the other. He is always hopeful that negotiation will take place, that people will "bend" a little and change, and that love will transcend all so that a consensus is reached. He believes that despite political power struggles and corruption, our democracy is based on good decisions being made most of the time and that one doesn't always have to be right. Lloyde declared that, "Even the most bashful, timid person could say something or comment on something and could very well influence as many as 10,000 people in their lives."

Lloyde has always enjoyed teaching, be it Sunday school or elementary school, to which he has devoted his professional life. He stresses the importance of educators, believing strongly that teachers should make every effort to reach children. "If we are going to influence society in a positive way, we have to do it through the children." According to Lloyde's philosophy, because no one method of teaching will work for every child, you have to start teaching children by finding out "where they are intellectually and advance them as far as you can." He also advocates educating parents along with their children, declaring that "ways must be developed to reach these families."

He grew up as the son of a minister and remembers his upbringing as stern and even harsh. His childhood was marked by many strict rules and corporal punishment. "My mother felt quite helpless and tried to be overly compassionate. I realized at a young age that there was much hypocrisy among people who professed to be religious."

Lloyde spoke at length about his late wife, Margaret. They met on a blind date and married when they both were about twenty-seven years old. Ironically, she lived across the street from him as they were growing up. They had two boys, and Lloyde asserted that his upbringing caused him to redouble his efforts to be more loving and understanding to his children. He loved

being a father and a husband, and adored and respected his wife dearly. Like her husband, Margaret was an elementary school teacher, and he felt she was one of the greatest teachers he had ever met. He said that kids, especially those with special needs, would flock to her because they felt that she not only cared about their learning things, but also cared about them as individuals. He believed that their marriage was so successful because they were completely honest with one another. They never misled one another or pretended. At the end of each day, Margaret would tell him what she had been thinking and he would share his thoughts with her. They lived in harmony and love. Lloyde and Margaret were married for twenty-five years before she died from cancer. He misses her terribly. "I have come to realize that I have developed a different kind of happiness in my life at the present time. I was truly happy with my wife, but I am also happy now and at peace."

When we asked Lloyde what he is most proud of and what evokes the most positive memories, he listed the following experiences: rooting for the Chicago Cubs; voting for Jimmy Carter; hearing FDR speak in the back of an observation car; and seeing Eleanor Roosevelt. She was rather homely, he admits, but once she spoke one never noticed her appearance.

"My only regret was being in the war. I couldn't find support to be a conscientious objector. My buddies could never convince me at all that war was necessary. It doesn't solve anything except that it sets it up for the next war." He believes that war is always civil war, because all are God's children. During the war he prayed to God to keep him alive, and his faith was strengthened. He felt that he could never shoot anyone, left his rifle against a tree, threw his gas mask away, and prayed to God. He was grateful that he did not have to go into combat and promised God that if he survived he would do something to serve mankind. He felt he was blessed to be assigned

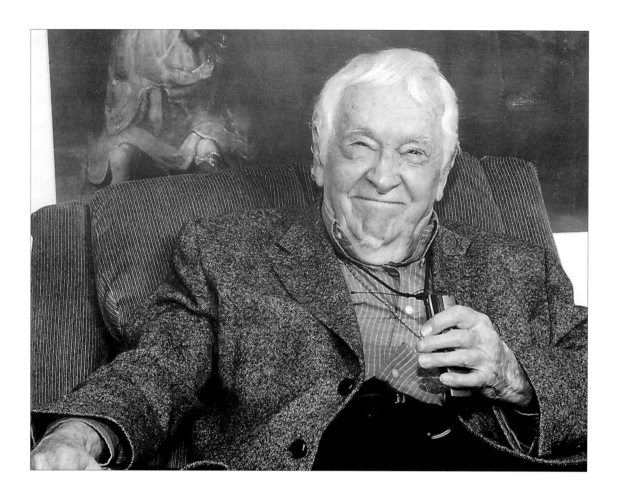

as a company clerk in the war, with typing as his main responsibility. When he returned to civilian life, he devoted the next few decades of his life to teaching children, and he now serves as a lay minister.

We asked Lloyde how he would advise this generation, and he pondered this question for several minutes. Emphasizing that a person's ideas about the world change almost daily, he replied, "This is a deeply involved question because it involves the generation finding out for themselves. I do feel that people try to search for happiness in things and stuff instead of really digging into our soul and feeling what is in each and every one of us if we take the time to feel."

BOB CHAMBERLIN

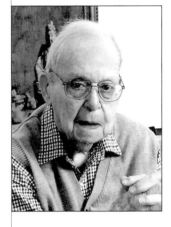

AGE: 98
"Live life to the fullest and enjoy every step of the way. Do your best and hope it comes out right."

"She loved this place." These simple words adorn a beautiful bronze plaque, mounted on a brick and limestone column at the entryway into the retirement village. This message honors Sue, Bob Chamberlin's late wife of sixty-eight years. After her death, Bob designed the plaque for Sue, who had loved every minute of her life at the retirement community. At ninety-eight, Bob confesses that the plaque really was created to comfort him in the loss of his beloved wife. However, the plaque has proved to be very popular among the residents, as demonstrated by the large crowd present for its dedication ceremony. It is gratifying to know that simplicity can be so meaningful and profound.

"Simplicity" was a theme that permeated our discussions with Bob. In talking about his marriage, he states that one of the high points of their marriage came in their early years, when they were living a simple life in which they fished and lived off the land. Bob's first job was in Bighorn Mountain, at a forest preserve 10,000-feet high. He and his wife lived there in a one-room cabin, and they both loved the challenge of the hard living conditions and primitive setting. He remembers that Sue learned to fly fish, and they ate fish almost every night. In a voice heavy with emotion, Bob states, "Fancy amenities don't make one happy. It was these simple times in nature that we treasured. My wife and I had a good marriage. It was based on mutual trust." He added, "I always had a feeling of satisfaction every day working with someone who sympathized, knew my high spots, and fed my low spots, which helped even things out. We each appreciated the other's interests." They loved and raised two children together, a son and daughter. "She brought a new perspective to my life coming from Europe. Sue was born and raised in France. Her father was a colonel in the French cavalry and, unfortunately, he died in the First World War. Sue's brother was a few years older than she, and her mother was terribly worried that he would

Authors' Reflection:
"Work to envelop nature into your days. It will nurture your soul throughout your life."

get drafted into the French army. All their kin had been in the army since Napoleonic days. Sue's mother completely uprooted her family, came to the United States, learned English, and established a life for her two children. Ultimately, Sue was the only heir remaining in her family, and she received a citation given to her great-great-great-grandfather, who was an officer with Napoleon in 1810 at the height of the latter's career. The citation reads that he was well recognized as a longtime and loyal citizen under Napoleon. This Legion of Honor award is like our Congressional Medal of Honor. Bob had it framed. Because the seal of Napoleon was so thick, they had to cut the glass from the frame.

Bob is very proud of Sue's many accomplishments. He explains that she was quite proficient in languages. He marvels at how, in her job at a bank, she could take dictation from the vice-president of foreign trade and translate it into French instantaneously. She would then retype it in English or Italian or German. Bob still has great appreciation and respect for his beloved late wife, and his memories of her and their life together clearly help to sustain him now that she is gone.

At ninety-eight years of age, Bob enjoyed reminiscing about his boyhood. He talked about growing up in Rochester, New York. "Rochester is known for heavy snow. If it is going to snow anywhere, it snows in Rochester and Buffalo which are ninety miles apart. I recall as a youngster going to elementary school in the winter. We would have to wait for the horse and plow to go through the sidewalks before we could start trudging to school. If the snow wasn't plowed, it was literally up to our hips. We all tried to wait until the plowman had come along. He would look like the 'Pied Piper' as all of us trudged along behind the plow. As kids we enjoyed inventing games to play. There was no television or radio, of course, just talkies." Bob also talked about his friends during that period and all that he learned from his scouting days. He feels the things he learned as a Boy Scout have carried him through his adulthood.

When we questioned Bob about his elementary and secondary education, he shared that he had had good teachers and was fortunate to have separate rooms for each grade even in the early nineteen hundreds. Ultimately, Bob earned a Bachelor of Landscape Architecture degree from the University of Michigan in 1931. He and his family were deeply affected by the Depression. His father was out of work, as were so many others. All needed money and were struggling simply to keep their homes and obtain enough food and gasoline. Bob stated, "It was a grim time for everybody." He chose to give up his graduate work and go to work to earn money for his family. It was fortuitous that his talents fit nicely with President Roosevelt's plan to "make work a program of worthwhile projects that are largely man built—not [built] by machine." He vividly remembers driving to a park and dropping off his father and another gentleman who had been a banker. These men were given a pick and shovel and put to work. Bob states that, in one way, the manual labor felt demeaning. Yet he remembers the sense of pride they felt in doing something for which they earned money and gained instant gratification from their efforts, instead of sitting at home ruminating over their misfortune. During the following years, President Roosevelt continued to expand existing parks and lay out new parks, thereby creating more jobs for people who needed them.

Bob moved back to Rochester, New York, and lived there many years. Rochester was considered "George Eastman Country." He had met George Eastman several times and enjoyed telling stories about him, even regarding him as his mentor. He recalled the time when the great industrialist bought the most expensive golf course in town. Bob described Eastman as an inventor and philanthropist, a nice and cordial man. His ideas generated jobs

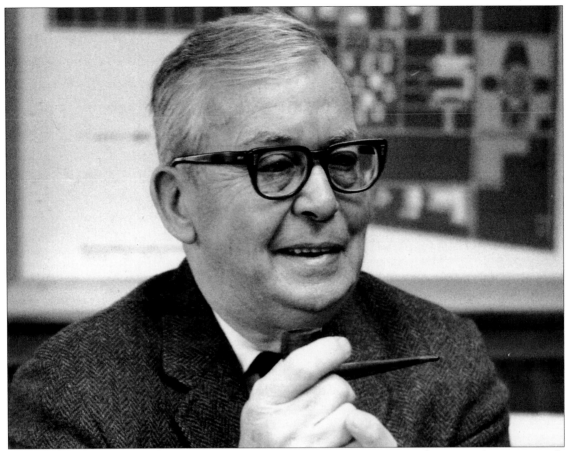

Bob enjoying his pipe at work.

for over half of the employees in the city of Rochester. When the Spanish influenza was killing people by the hundreds, George Eastman knew that children who still had their adenoids and tonsils might be saved if they were removed. As a philanthropist, he offered to pay for the operation for every affected child in the city of Rochester. Mr. Eastman also loved music and offered to buy an instrument for every child who wished to play one. His only requirement was that the student practice and become somewhat proficient. As so many people are aware, he built the prestigious Eastman School of Music in Rochester on a site surrounded by huge oak trees and the river. With painful disbelief, Bob recalls that when Mr. Eastman had accomplished all he had set out to do, he went upstairs, and left a note that read, "My work is done, Why wait?" and shot himself.

Eastman's life had a profound effect on Bob. He decided to leave his own legacy through his love of landscaping. In his career as a landscape architect, Bob always strived to help buildings "come alive" by surrounding them with living things. He converted an enormous piece of barren land, originally corn and soybean fields, into twenty-eight acres of inviting living space. Over this acreage, he created intimate areas where people might read, rest, or contemplate. When he and others planted the trees—a labor of love that Bob fondly remembers—they were two inches in diameter. Now they are over a foot in diameter, and he is delighted when he sees people enjoying the picnic areas he envisioned in the early stages of his planning. Bob also designed areas that attracted many different types of birds. This developed land was the site of what ultimately became Bob and Sue's retirement village. Bob realized early in his life how important it was to have "outside" rooms that reflected one's mood and enhanced one's appreciation of nature as a part of everyday life.

After a long career as a landscape architect, Bob wanted to share his favorite selection of trees. He has always appreciated the beauty and majesty of trees. One of his favorite species is the white redbud, "An anomaly of sorts," he points out, "but they are sensational." In his work, he often included designs for crabapple trees, as they come in so many different colors and shades. They also last longer so people can thoroughly enjoy them. Among the maple trees, Bob enjoys the "Red Sunset" most because of its brilliant red color in the fall. His two other favorites are the gingko and beech trees. Each has held special significance for him during his life. The gingko has been around since the time of the dinosaurs, and it is totally different from other trees. Its leaves are shaped like little fans and are heavily veined and

leathery to the touch. The trees turn a bright gold color and drop their leaves all at once. One can easily sense Bob's appreciation for this "historical and unique specimen." A purple beech tree currently is positioned right in front of Bob's living-room window. This has special meaning, as it was planted in his honor when he retired from his University of Illinois position in 1971. He also has a special bird feeder in full view. He quipped that he may have to put up a sign inviting the birds as he hasn't seen many visitors lately.

Bob's advice to everyone is to "Live life to the fullest and enjoy every step of the way. Do your best and hope it comes out right. Surround yourself with people who have the same interests and values." We asked Bob to what he attributed his longevity, and he quickly responded: "Abstaining from cigarettes (although I smoked a pipe most of my life), being happily married, and being able to do what I loved—landscaping. I made a lot of friends who initially were clients. I learned what each client liked—trees, flowers, and other interesting vegetation." Bob admits that he loves old movies and all documentaries about the time between 1910 and 1920. Bob likes CNN and enjoys checking his e-mail for correspondence from his two children. He also did crossword puzzles until very recently. He particularly enjoyed the *New York Times* puzzles. Bob continues to read novels. Recently, he has been rereading a book on Abraham Lincoln. He comments that President Lincoln "not only was brilliant, but also must have been a man of great character. Most great men are." Bob's advice to young people is to obtain an education to the limit that they can afford.

His only lament is, "It is so sad that war still continues. I do have guilt that I didn't serve in World War II. Because I had an education, I needed to stay in the U.S. and train men in different capacities. The University of Illinois was set up as a Navy Signal Corps for diesel school training where young men learned to be signalmen. During lunchtime, all the men marched and sang patriotic songs. People in the streets and others looking out the windows would look forward to the noon experience. Although Bob knew that he and the other men were providing a necessary service, he still felt that he needed to always explain why he wasn't in the war. "This war we are in now concerns me.... War is a waste, and it is a shame that we cannot talk and live together in peace."

MABEL JONES

When we first met Mabel Jones she was sitting in her colorful, crisply ironed dress, her crossword puzzles and hometown newspaper close at hand. She put us completely at ease as we began our interview.

Ninety-six-year-old Mabel has enjoyed a long life marked by an abiding love for language. Whether through reading a good newspaper story, mastering a crossword puzzle, engaging in a rousing conversation, or composing poetry, language has been Mabel's primary and most pleasing way to stay connected to her world.

Mabel admits her pleasure in doing crossword puzzles, with only her magnifying glass to aid her. She often works on the puzzles while watching her favorite shows, "Jeopardy" and "Wheel of Fortune." One of the highlights of each day continues to be going to the mailbox for her newspaper. She always stacks the newspapers on the porch, and her daughter knows that it is important never to throw them away until Mabel herself places them in a different part of the room.

Language in the form of poetry has been a joy and comfort throughout her life. She began memorizing poems as a young child as a challenge. From the time she was very young, she has relied on writing poetry to express her feelings and emotions.

After Mabel had read some of her poetry to us during one of our interviews, she shared some details of her life. She was married when she was eighteen years old to her high school sweetheart. Although she didn't finish high school, Mabel attended a night school where she learned to type and take shorthand. She passed with flying colors and proudly received two certificates. Unfortunately, being black made it difficult for her to get a job. More sad times ensued as Mabel's husband left her when her two young daughters were in preschool. She was forced to move back in with her mother and father. Perseverance was a trademark of hers, and she began

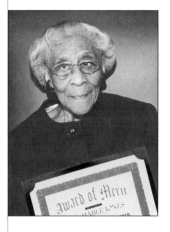

AGE: 96

"It isn't the house alone that makes a home. It is the 'family' that dwells within."

Authors' Reflection:
"Persevere in spite of racism and sexism. With those evils confronted, life is worth living."

85

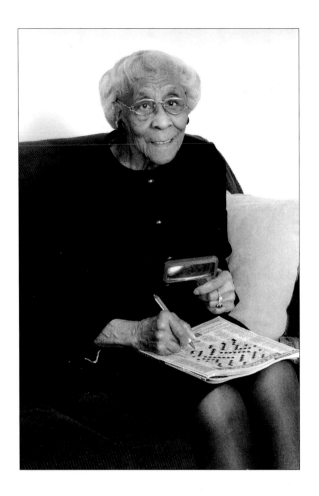

working with the WPA (Works Progress Administration), which had been initiated by President Roosevelt. She sewed clothing for people on "relief," a government assistance program that is comparable to our present welfare system. Later, Mabel performed housekeeping duties at a hospital. Her next position, and the one she loved, was at Williamson Press Company in Springfield, Illinois. She fondly remembers three business partners for whom she worked for thirty-two years. Although they were white men and it was a time when the rights of African-Americans were not protected by law, Mabel remembers how they valued her as a human being. They considered themselves "family." She vividly recalled her first assignment wrapping packages by hand with her bosses nearby. Later, they all worked together to print menus, books, and forms. When the business grew and moved to a more desirable location, Mabel composed a poem and placed a copy on each of their desks. Each verse begins with the first letter of their names. The poem had not been seen in a long time, when Mabel's daughter, Florence, suddenly came upon it in Mabel's bedroom one day.

The Three

Looking far into the future
Upward now we climb
Every step gets smoother
Rough roads are left behind.

Don't awaken me if I am…
Our faces with smiles are beaming
Relieved from the traffic jam
Restricted areas are all around.

Stairways have all been "erased"
Measures 30,000 feet all on the ground
It is a wonderful place!
Time marches on at W.P.I.
Hats off, "The Three" are passing by.
Mabel 1-17-57

Mabel confided that the men were greatly touched by the poem she wrote in honor of their working relationship and friendship. However, she was humble about her motivation, stating, "I would like to toss a bouquet to 'The Three' of Williamson Press, Inc. I feel that they had the vision to look far ahead into

the future, and see the need for purchasing a building suitable for the housing and operation of the printing business. They are to be commended!" Mabel greatly enjoyed the comfort and amenities of the new building. However, with deep feeling, Mabel expressed what the move really meant to her: "It isn't the house alone that makes a home. It is the 'family' that dwells within. The only thing we left at 221 South Fourth Street [old location] was the building. We moved all of our 'furniture' and the family was still intact. Now, more so than ever before, we were together as one, big family and could all work together for the betterment of the business."

Speaking of her early life, Mabel recalled that her father was a minister and that both her parents had founded the Grace United Methodist Church in Springfield, Illinois. As the youngest of five children, she takes pride in remembering that she "didn't get paddled as much as her older siblings." Mabel can recall all of the addresses of her past homes, something "most people my age can't do." She remembers fondly her family's living in a two-story home, with beautiful hedges and a fence. There were also three porches, located on the front, side, and back of the home, evoking memories of a time when people knew their neighbors and met on the porch to sip lemonade and talk. Mabel became quite animated when she described her family's indoor plumbing and telephone. Reflecting on the household of her youth, Mabel commented that her father didn't approve of "fussin' and cussin'," and declared, "You children should know what to say by what I say." Although Mabel's father professed not to allow "cussin'," one exception was Aunt Julia, who came to visit bearing the most delicious homemade pies and cakes, but who also would cuss. Mabel's father excused it for Julia's sake because she had a good heart.

Mabel's faith and connections to her church have always been important in her life. She is proud to say that her minister from Springfield,

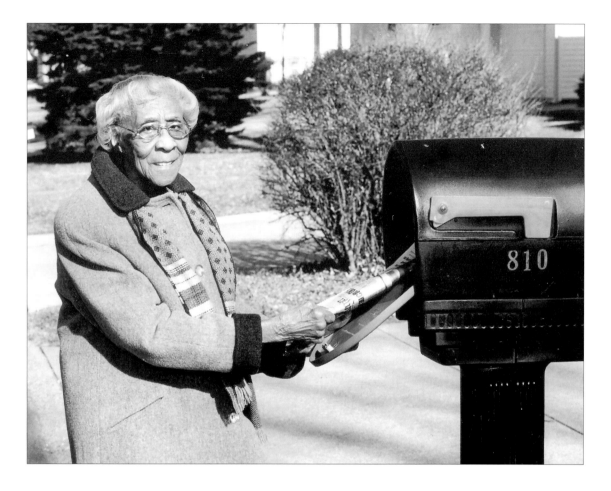

Illinois continued to visit her even after she moved 100 miles away. Mabel remembers enjoying hearing her old minister bring her news of the people she knew who still lived in Springfield. She relates how, on one visit, the minister brought her a plaque commemorating her as the oldest member of the church and had her photographed holding the plaque. As the picture was about to be taken, Mabel recalls that her daughter pointed out that the plaque looked crooked. Mabel immediately quipped, "It may be crooked, but I'm not a crook!"

Although she is ninety-six years old, Mabel has strong opinions about contemporary society. She is convinced that the young girls in the twenty-first

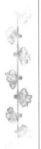

century would be more attractive if they covered up. Mabel laughingly states, "If you girls want to show yourselves, stay home and get naked." She attributes her longevity to genes and to luck. She never smoked or drank, except once in a while, socially, when she didn't want other women to think she was arrogant. Mabel always had well-manicured nails, and her friends teased her saying she had false nails. Mabel replied, "Nothing about me is fake."

Mabel states that she has been inspired by certain sayings all of her life: "Don't let anyone talk you into doing something you are not comfortable with." "Be who you are." "Don't feel ashamed to ask if you don't know something." "If you can't fix a situation, don't worry about it." "To each his own." "DON'T JUDGE." "Sometimes friends are family." "It needs to be like that and has to be like that." Mabel treated us to one of her own quotes when Chuck, the photographer, was about to take her picture. Ninety-six-year-old Mabel, sitting in front of her hutch full of old treasures, smiled up at Chuck and said, "Should I say sex or cheese?"

Note: February 5, 2006
Kim called tonight and told me that Mabel had died. How could we mourn and grieve for a woman we hardly knew? Florence, Mabel's daughter, shared that her mother started acting differently a few weeks before she died. Mabel started getting into boxes that were in her bedroom that contained obituaries of friends and loved ones who had passed away. Her daughter thinks it was because she knew she would be seeing them soon. When Mabel died, Florence said she had the most peaceful smile on her face. Mabel had touched our hearts, and we felt we would give anything for a few more minutes to savor her sweetness, candor, poetic side, sentimental nature, and lovely spirit. Kim sat with Mabel a week before she died and recorded her low voice reciting a poem she had remembered about being

honest with oneself. With poignant intensity, Mabel's voice intoned the following insightful guide to living with responsibility and honor. It is based on Edgar Guest's poem "Myself."

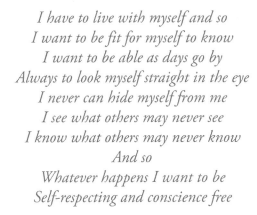

I have to live with myself and so
I want to be fit for myself to know
I want to be able as days go by
Always to look myself straight in the eye
I never can hide myself from me
I see what others may never see
I know what others may never know
And so
Whatever happens I want to be
Self-respecting and conscience free

BERNICE HAWBAKER

Bernice Hawbaker epitomizes the meaning behind the phrase "a life well spent." At 104 years of age, Bernice still enjoys a rich and interesting life. She resides with her three devoted daughters, rotating every two weeks from one home to the next. One of these homes sits in the lovely country-side near where she spent much of her life, and the other two are in cities nearby.

Bernice starts each morning by making her own bed. She then fixes her breakfast, which always includes a biscuit, some homemade peach butter, and some sausage or bacon. She always takes a fifteen-minute walk at some point during the day, with one of her daughters at her side. Bernice loves to read, especially "love stories." Her daughter Joanie reports that she recently read three books in two weeks. She takes a nap every afternoon, a tradition that has been part of her life since her children were little. Bernice enjoys TV, especially John Wayne movies and family shows like reruns of the "Waltons." A favorite outing for her is going with family members for pizza, or to a local buffet that features food prepared by the Amish.

Until very recently, Bernice crocheted beautiful doilies and tablecloths. Her many finished products are true works of art—intricate, graceful, and a reminder of her love to all of her family and friends who have received them as gifts. Over the years, she has included her crocheted doilies in the cards she sent out for birthdays, holidays, or other special occasions. Bernice also loved making crocheted crosses for acquaintances she met who shared her religious faith.

This loving gesture of sharing with others has carried over into other realms of her life. Joanie comments that her mother has always given gifts of fruit from her strawberry patch and fruit trees, along with her homemade cobblers, pies, and noodles. In fact, until she reached 103 years of age, Bernice still made homemade noodles and cobblers for all family gatherings

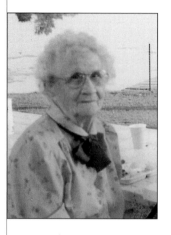

AGE: 104

"Meat, butter, and cow's milk—these were good eats."

Authors' Reflection:
"Meaningful traditions make lasting impressions and generational memories."

93

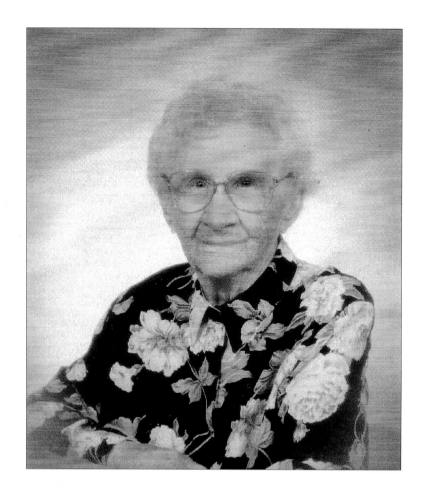

and gained much notoriety among admirers for her wonderful cooking. She recalls that her mother has always recognized the needs of her family, friends, and neighbors, adding, "My mother always helped the underdog and gave of herself even when she didn't have much material wealth to share."

One of Bernice's favorite and most cherished recipes among her family members is for "Grandma's Noodles":

Grandma's Noodles

Beat 2 eggs; add 2 tablespoons cream or milk and 1 scant teaspoon of salt. Add enough flour (2/3 to 1 cup) to make a soft dough. Roll paper-thin and let dry. Cut fine and add to boiling broth. Cook 15 to 30 minutes, stirring often to prevent sticking. To increase this portion, add 1 egg, 1 tablespoon cream or milk, 1/8 teaspoon salt, and 2/3 cup flour.

Bernice looks back on a full, rich life. She admits that what she misses most about her past is her husband; they had been married sixty-two years when he died. Bernice states, "I miss my husband terribly. We shared a lot of great times together. I still remember the first horses we rode together!" She continues, "I miss my vegetable and flower gardens. I really miss my gladiolas—they are my favorite." Still sharing her gifts and secrets, Bernice notes, "I don't think people should use tap water when watering their flowers. For great big blooms that will double in size and beauty, I recommend treating once a month with the following:

1 gallon tepid water,

1 teaspoon baking powder,

1 teaspoon Epsom salt,

1 teaspoon saltpeter, and

1/8 teaspoon household ammonia."

Summertime always reminds Bernice of how she loved going to the old Fourth of July celebrations, which included a special yearly picnic near their home. The family would sit on the grass to eat, visit with others, and watch people get shot out of a cannon! Bernice also has many wonderful memories about her parents. Her mother was a teacher and also a great cook who made delicious homemade treats for her family. With a twinkle in her eye, Bernice states that she can still taste her mother's gingerbread and the fancy cakes that stood proudly on her Mother's elegant cake stand. She recalls the layers of icing her mother always made and the famous Texas sheet cake that her mother baked every year for Bernice's birthday (with walnuts picked from the family walnut tree, of course). Another birthday treat was a watermelon given to her each year by her dad—during the month of the

year that watermelons were at their best. She recalls her mother's cooking reflected living off the land, and adds with a laugh, "Meat, butter, and cow's milk—these were good eats."

Bernice Hawbaker, now a centenarian, is still living her life as a long-time beloved mother, grandmother, and faithful friend. She had three daughters and one son. At the age of 104, she still takes great pleasure in admiring pictures of her grandchildren and great-grandchildren. She enjoys passing on advice about where to purchase a particularly beautiful variety of African violet, a plant that she saw recently for the first time. She lives her life simply and with appreciation, providing a good role model for those around her. Others can learn from her life that the memories that sustain us are never related to wealth, status, or prestige. Love expressed in terms of nurturing another's spirit, feeding our souls with handmade "acts of kindness," taking time to enjoy nature, living in the moment, anticipating the needs of others, never forgetting the simple graces and dignities of life, appreciating and nurturing all the people who are important in our existence—these are the ways that Bernice has thrived in her "life well spent." In honor of Bernice's 100th birthday, her siblings, children, grandchildren, and great-grandchildren presented a book compiled of letters, poems, and pictures that reflected memories of their time spent with her. One memorable letter and poem follows:

Dear Grandma,

Visiting you has always been wonderful. My first memories are of you in the gray farmhouse. I remember a back porch full of kittens eating leftovers from a pie pan. We sat on the steps by the garden to break beans and shell peas. You had a full-time job just cooking and cleaning up meals, but you always had time to play cards, marbles or teach me to crochet. Many times you were very patient as I tagged along wanting to be a part of everything you did.

Many times cousins would come and then the peaceful countryside turned into anything young minds could imagine. You gave us dishes to play restaurant in the shed. We were cowboys and Indians in the pasture; we played tag until exhaustion, told ghost stories in every scary location we could find, and acted like Tarzan and Jane in the barn. Someone always got hurt! There were splinters, falls, broken glass and legs coming through the ceiling. You always remained calm. As I got older and you moved to Dunn Station, our time together changed. I became much more interested in your recipes, handwork quilting and green thumb flowers. We have shared those same interests for many years.

I cherish those memories of visiting you and I pray there are many more to come. Enjoy this remarkable birthday.

I love you!
Donna

In Memory of the "Home Place"

Sold At Auction February 25, 1993
Farm for Sale
Just an empty house
Where people live no more.
Broken dreams and windows
Rusty hinges on the door.

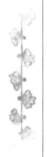

Memories in every corner
Where spiders now call home.
Silent footsteps on the stairs
Where have the children gone?

Shadows hug the garden
Where babies used to play
Wild flowers nod and whisper
As they speak of yesterday.

The pine tree cries in agony
Upon his chest A Nail!
Holding up a sign that says
"This House and Farm for Sale."
(By Iris, daughter)

Note:
Bernice Hawbaker passed away peacefully on October 2, 2006.

Leave Your Legacy

LEAVE YOUR LEGACY

A legacy is one of the most precious gifts you can leave your children, grand-children and other loved ones. It will provide a way of sharing advice and practical information that could be of great benefit to others.

CHILDHOOD

What was your childhood home and neighborhood like?

What did you admire most about your parents?

What did you learn from your parents?

How did you get along with your siblings, and how has your relationship changed through the years?

What were the happiest times of your childhood?

Other than family, who were the most important people in your life when you were growing up?

What were your childhood friends like? What types of activities did you do for fun?

What do you remember most vividly regarding your school experiences from elementary through high school?

What traditions and holiday memories do you cherish?

What was the most mischievous thing you did as a child?

ADULTHOOD: LOVE AND FAMILY

What do you think are the secrets to a good marriage or relationship?

What is your definition of love? Have your thoughts changed over the years?

What was the best time you had as a family?

What do you remember being the hardest time you had as a family?

Which family vacation was your favorite?

What was the most rewarding aspect of raising kids? What was the most difficult aspect of raising kids?

Do you have any advice about being a good parent?

THINGS I HAVE ENJOYED

Do you have a favorite book or author?

List some of your favorite movies?

What are some of your favorite foods?

Do you have any family recipes you would like to share?

THOUGHTS AND REFLECTIONS

What were the best years of your life?

What do you think are the most important things in life?

Do you believe in God?

Do you think life now is harder or easier than when you were growing up?

What are you most proud of?

What do you think is the secret to a long-lasting friendship?

How would you like to be remembered?